Human Side of a Surgeon

For

Maryanne

enjoy

H. Ballentield

HUMAN SIDE OF A SURGEON

Harold Battenfield

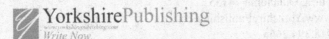

YorkshirePublishing
www.yorkshirepublishing.com
Write Now.

Yorkshire Publishing
3207 South Norwood Avenue
Tulsa, Oklahoma 74135
www.YorkshirePublishing.com
918.394.2665

For Mary

Who believed in me before I dared to believe in myself

CONTENTS

Preface ix

The Education of a Surgeon

CHAPTER 1   1955-1965 1
CHAPTER 2   1965-1968 13

The Life of a Surgeon

CHAPTER 3   1968-1974 49
CHAPTER 4   1975 67
CHAPTER 5   1976-1987 85
CHAPTER 6   1988-2010 115
CHAPTER 7   Collected Stories from the ER 129
CHAPTER 8   Reflections: 2010-2017 145

PREFACE

At thirty I was aware of my lack of experience and patience. Anxious to prove myself to the two orthopedic surgeons whose practice I had joined, I tried to measure my words and maintain good eye contact with patients, wanting them to understand I was concerned and attentive to their needs.

On my second day of practice, a sixty-year-old man with knee pain sat on the examining table in my office. Wanting to sit down on the rolling stool behind me without losing eye contact, I took two steps backward. In one fluid motion smoother than a circus act, my heel pushed down on the foot pedal of the trashcan, the lid lifted, and in I fell.

Red-faced, I scrambled onto the stool, hoping my patient hadn't noticed the obvious.

Breaking into a belly laugh he said, "My wife's not going to believe me."

Though I can't recall actual dialogue through the years, I am comfortable filling in the spaces. The intent is true. I enjoy stories about my profession, particularly when they involve doctors who worked on the frontier of orthopedic surgery. Previous generations of surgeons made mistakes and we who stood on their shoulders benefitted from their errors, as did our profession.

Great books on surgery do exist, even a few orthopedic surgery texts, but not one has ever made me laugh. These books didn't explore the dark side of our profession, explaining what went wrong in a procedure. Typical autobiographies written by surgeons certainly haven't delved into the emotional life of a surgeon. The books were rational, implying that if a doctor followed the rules, all would turn out well. I could sanitize my words at the cost of not telling the truth, but I won't.

Much of this book is subjective, but so is life. Wisdom comes from experience gleaned through practice, patience, and pain. The tuition is high.

Frequently an orthopedic surgeon practiced within the constraints of modern medicine in communities without peers for consultation, and he had to innovate with the crude, limited tools at hand. We considered unusual encounters the norm. I've attempted to convey this sense of isolation. I value the necessity for physicians to follow established protocols and culture that culminate in the official version of facts. Professional journals condense studies into objective results and outcomes. However, members of our profession often sidestepped isolated errors and unusual experiences that became the in-the-closet truths. I experienced many surprises in my medical career, and my intent is to address them within a spirit of caring, no matter how comical they may have been. Stories both sad and humorous were all in a day's work and often illustrated a level of compassion on the part of a doctor that the public never witnessed.

For simplicity, I refer to the surgeon as *he* while recognizing female orthopedic surgeons abound in practice today. Although the medical community uses the metric system, I have used the imperial because it's more common in the U.S.

During my professional life, I was sometimes the teacher and sometimes the student. That was as good as it gets and I was blessed. For my part in this professional world, I carry the responsibility of saving the history of progress as I experienced it. My experiences led to my maturation as a resident physician, orthopedic surgeon, husband, father, and grandfather. These roles and events in my life braided together and formed my character.

This book is true except for the parts I embellished.

H. B.

THE EDUCATION OF A SURGEON

1955-1968

NORTHEASTERN STATE UNIVERSITY
OKLAHOMA
Four Years Undergraduate

BACHELOR DEGREE

KANSAS CITY UNIVERSITY
OF MEDICINE AND BIOSCIENCE
Four Years Medical School

DOCTOR OF OSTEOPATHIC MEDICINE

OKLAHOMA OSTEOPATHIC HOSPITAL
One-year Primary Care Internship

LICENSE TO PRACTICE MEDICINE

KANSAS CITY UNIVERSITY
OF MEDICINE AND BIOSCIENCE
Four Years Orthopedic Residency

ORTHOPEDIC SURGEON

CHAPTER 1

NORTHEASTERN STATE UNIVERSITY
1955-1959

World War II and the Korean Conflict closed the era of my coming of age. The average young man graduating from high school in my era could count on working indefinitely in the same field which would develop as our country expanded. Growing up in Muskogee, Oklahoma, I functioned in an environment of limited competition, but I didn't know it.

My college experience in Tahlequah, Oklahoma provided an awakening to options in the world. My first college class was accounting. I didn't care for it, so I drifted back into chemistry where I had worked as an assistant in the chemistry lab in high school during my senior year. I liked that chemistry tied into physics and mathematics. My grades were good so I visited two pre-med meetings, but I was too insecure to go public and say I was pre-med. The brother of my girlfriend Mary was two years into medical school in Kansas City and invited me to visit. As a profession and as individuals, the medical school gave me a grand tour and made me feel welcome. From the school's perspective, if students had the grades to be accepted, it was the school's responsibility to help them graduate.

When I applied to medical school, over half of the potential competing students did not apply. Females and African Americans constituted less than five percent of my class.

During the spring of my senior year at Northeastern State University in Tahlequah OK, I received notice of admittance to Kansas City

1

University of Medicine and Biosciences for the fall semester. I was also informed a $220 deposit was required to hold my position. I had $220 like I had extra teeth to sell. Because my parents didn't even understand why I went to college, asking them for financial help for medical school was not an option.

With her senior year at NSU still ahead, Mary planned to attend summer school and receive her teaching degree by the end of the fall semester. She came to my rescue by giving her dorm deposit to secure my place.

"I can live there at least a month before they kick me out," she said, her eyes twinkling with mischief.

By working at a lumberyard and selling my shotgun, I reimbursed her the week she moved into the dorm.

KANSAS ITY UNIVERSITY OF MEDICINE AND BIOSCIENCES

1959-1963

I anticipated having much in common with fellow students. However, my class of 107 was a cross-section of cultures from around the country: nine religions, three African-Americans, four females, and several older students. The older students brought broader life experiences to the group, particularly five pharmacists who possessed less-rigid opinions and showed tolerance for opposing views. Their maturity influenced the group's behavior.

As I shed the limitations of my perspectives, I learned from those around me. Easterners spoke in rapid-fire fashion and I learned to think faster to follow along. On the other hand, they had to slow down and listen closely to understand my Oklahoma drawl. Much later I came to appreciate the varied personalities and values of the other students. Diversity delivered value.

On our first day of anatomy class, we filed into the lab room without talking. A towel had been placed over each cadaver's face. The proctor explained that not seeing the anonymous person on the table provided time for adjustment. He further assigned four students to each table with a cadaver. We found ourselves whispering. Our proctor stood silent for what felt like hours until our whispering ceased.

"We expect you to value the people lying on the table in front of you. All were volunteers to be on this table for you. For this we thank them."

His words permeated the room like a prayer. "Do not give them names."

The following week the towels were no longer needed.

The next week we stood around the cadaver table grilling each other on anatomical terms: biceps, triceps, radius, ulna, etc. A tablemate would pick up a tendon and ask the name and receive a quick response, "*Sartorius*." Another placed his index finger under a muscle above the patella. "What's the name of this one?" The fellow next to me said, "*Vastus lateralus*."

I thought he was wrong, but I didn't respond. I spoke only when I was sure my answer was correct, fearing everyone else knew anatomy better than me.

By the end of the second week, I felt I didn't have any business being in medical school. I planned to take the first examination during the fourth week and go home. To my astonishment I scored the highest grade at our table, a defining moment in my life. Realizing my tablemates had been guessing at answers, I determined never to pretend I knew something when I didn't. I never again let the words "I don't know" hang in my throat.

Thereafter, I questioned anyone who appeared to always have an answer.

~~~

Mary graduated from college mid-year, and we were married over the Christmas holiday. She began teaching first grade in the Kansas City public school system. Because males were considered the heads of their households, they received five hundred dollars more than female teachers. Mary was our breadwinner but not considered head of household even though I was unemployed. We relied on what she earned.

Medical students of this era were required, under supervision, to oversee three pregnancies to term before graduation to ensure a foundation in obstetrics.

My first patient was an 18-year-old less nervous than I. When she realized she was my first, she patted the back of my hand and counseled me with a soothing voice. Throughout the appointments for her pregnancy we conversed, and by the time of her successful delivery, we had developed a friendship. Our bonding resulted in a decades-long association of exchanging Christmas cards, even years after she became a grandmother.

The two remaining pregnancies under my care delivered without problems, leading me to assume all others would happen in a like manner. In the event of a complicated case, I figured consulting staff stood by to assist.

OKLAHOMA OSTEOPATHIC HOSPITAL
1963-1964

After graduation in 1963, I wrestled with the direction my life should take. I spent a year interning at Oklahoma Osteopathic Hospital in Tulsa, later to become Oklahoma State Medical Center. I rotated through the four specialties, each for three months: surgery, emergency room, obstetrics, and internal medicine. The attending physicians were appropriately friendly and tolerated students looking over their shoulders while they answered our simple questions.

I had read a medical journal that advised students not to confuse any specialty with a dynamic personality in the field, but one attending physician during my internship was different from the others. An orthopedic surgeon named Dr. Felmlee asked our names and seemed genuinely interested in us as people, as opposed to badgering us as students.

I equated Dr. Felmlee with orthopedics and therefore chose orthopedics as my speciality.

The closest hospitals with orthopedic training programs were in Kansas City and Dayton. Competition was intense. I'd already invested four years in medical school, one year in rotating internship to obtain my license to practice, and now I was considering adding four more years.

Well-meaning friends and relatives asked me about my plans. Not wanting to be embarrassed, I kept responses short and vague. I didn't want to apply to a specialty, be rejected, and then have to explain to everyone. I fretted about what Mary really wanted and what would be best for our one-year-old daughter Lori.

In the weeks that followed, I listened when older staff members talked about politics, government, and their general plans in the lunchroom. When they discussed their lives, I leaned in, alert for pointers because I was about to make a lifetime decision. One particular table became my favorite.

"I wish I had gone into a radiology residency right out of internship," said one doctor in the lunchroom who looked to be in his thirties. "I figured I'd work a few years in family practice while I paid off my debts and then decide," he continued. "Before I knew it, our kids were in school and my wife loved the neighbors and the church."

Taking the doctor's story to heart, I vowed not to go into debt setting up my own practice and looked for a salaried job near Tulsa since I hadn't heard from any of the orthopedic programs.

After passing the licensing exam, I needed to make my decision. I vowed not to go into debt setting up my own practice and instead looked for a salaried job near Tulsa. I located a primary care physician named Dr. Knight practicing in Houston who was so busy he wanted to open a satellite office. I landed the job over the phone and he offered to subsidize me. With his guidance and used furniture, I set up a small office two miles down the road from his without having to go into debt. He understood that if a position opened in Kansas City for a four-year residency in orthopedic surgery, I would leave. I soon learned a new office was a slow-growth business and looked for additional income.

"Dr. Buckner could use some help in Houston and there's not much paperwork," Knight said one day.

PRIMARY CARE PRACTICE
1964-1965

Dr. Buckner's office was in Houston's ghetto. Two lawn chairs welcomed me in the reception area where a simple placard on the wall announced, "Cash Only." I had seen more decorations in an elevator. Across the room, a middle-aged guy sat smoking in a rocking chair behind a card-table desk. A ceramic bowl rested on the floor for ashes.

A nurse called me back to Buckner's office. He sat behind a roll-top desk on a stool with a Post Toasties calendar on the wall behind his head.

We chatted. His busy day practice included daytime deliveries. He needed another doctor to deliver babies at night. His fee of $240 covered two office calls, lab work, delivery, and a 24-hour stay in his hospital across the street. He owned a house that served as a licensed hospital before local and federal regulations required otherwise.

He contracted with me to deliver babies at night for $40 per delivery, warning that after eight o'clock in the evening there was no guarantee of having a nurse to assist me.

"I can do that," I said, as though I had delivered hundreds.

"Want to start today?" He turned to the wall calendar and scribbled in my name. "If I don't take care of these folks, nobody will. I know the people and ghetto well. Been here fifteen years. They know the rules. My collections are one hundred percent and my office call is three dollars. Once upon a time I gave credit and then everyone expected it."

I perched on the edge of my chair alternately dumbfounded and impressed.

"Once upon a time I gave credit and then everyone expected it. I went broke. Now I don't even give credit for an injection of penicillin. Patients pay the nurse and then the nurse gives the injection."

He studied my face for a few moments, and I knew he was gauging my reaction.

"No one is offended. I provide a service no one else can."

Without a written agreement or signature, we shook hands.

Buckner was not a character but a doctor with character and strong values. Other doctors referred to him as the "missionary doctor." He practiced with the idealism of a missionary. His sincerity impressed me and I liked him.

He didn't have a reception desk and his only help was a part-time, untrained nurse. Despite dealing in cash only, his income fell well below the average. He kept his medical records on three-by-five cards. I soon understood his patients were not run-of-the-mill or average people, but people locked into poverty and ignorance.

Our telephone rang at one-thirty in the morning, calling me to my first delivery, one without supervisions or an anesthesiologist.

I pulled into a gravel parking lot across from Buckner's office, turned off the ignition, and took a deep breath. Leaning into the windshield, I eyed the four-hundred-square-foot house. The word "hospital" was handwritten vertically on a one-by-four post driven into the front yard. An old swing on the front porch hung motionless in the sweltering night air of Houston in July.

When I walked through the door, Eleanor was busy tending two patients and manning the barred admissions window. Not certified as a nurse but qualified with thirty years of on-the-job training, Eleanor functioned at night as bookkeeper, nurse, midwife, janitor, laundress, and maintenance man. She wore shorts because of the undependable window air conditioning. Regardless of how she dressed on the job, she was the boss. When she talked, I listened.

A woman clearly having contractions stood on the other side of the bars.

"Justine," Eleanor said to her, "I see by your chart you haven't paid in full. You owe thirty dollars." The woman started to protest but stopped herself and waddled out of the building.

"You can't turn her away," I scolded.

"I think I just did." Eleanor flipped her wrist. "She knew the rules. She's bluffing. Watch her parked car. She'll either sit there and have a few more contractions or she'll leave and come back with the money. Justine wouldn't have come in in the first place if she didn't have the money." She motioned toward my patient. "You need to take care of

Lettie. She was dilated four centimeters when I called you and should be at least eight or nine by now. By the way, what did you say your name was?"

"Dr. Battenfield."

"Well, Battenfield, you take care of your patient and I'll handle the parking-lot lady."

The house boasted three tiny bedrooms, two for labor and one for delivery, the latter with a sheet hung over the single window to block the view of curious family members standing in the backyard. In good weather, the sheet could be pulled back and hung on a nail to permit ventilation. All interior doors, except for the bathroom, had been removed to benefit from the single inadequate window AC. One toilet served everyone.

Good-natured Lettie, whose water had broken, weighed 242 pounds. To keep cool in the humid air, she wore only a red bib apron with "Kiss the Cook" scrolled across the top in yellow. As this was her eighth delivery, she calmly informed me a neighbor had dropped her off and would pick her up the following day.

Between Lettie's contractions, I periodically looked out the front window to check on Justine, who remained sitting in her car in the parking lot. I shook my head. I didn't understand the system.

Lettie moaned as her labor advanced.

With both of us grunting and groaning, she stepped up on a stool and I scooted her butt onto the delivery table. I felt as if I were tussling with a waterbed. We settled her body parts on the table one lump at a time. Only one of the table's thigh straps functioned, so I secured her other foot to the stirrup with adhesive tape. I intended to use my own belt as a backup plan.

Without an anesthesiologist to administer more advanced medication, I injected a much less effective local anesthetic to the nerve fibers that supply the muscles and skin in the vaginal area. I injected more around her vagina and, not sure how much I had injected, made a third pass.

"You're doin' fine, doc—*grunt*—just hang in there—*grunt*—we're gonna birth this baby," Lettie said between contractions. Despite more time and encouragement, she was not progressing.

I grew concerned and didn't know what to do next. It was now 2:30 a.m. My hands trembled, and my voice shook. I was alone and afraid with no one to call for help and no hospital to accept her.

"Doc—*grunt*—I've had eight babies and never been on my back 'cept to get pregnant—*grunt*—so if you untie my feet and help me down, I can do this."

I stared at her.

"Listen to me! Just untie my feet—*grunt*—and help me down!"

Perhaps she was going to leave and I wouldn't have blamed her. I kind of wished she would.

"I never had a baby on my back before and it don't feel right. I need to hang onto this table leg and squat. Like taking a shit."

Because Lettie had a plan and I didn't, I released her legs. With her arms around my neck, I sat her up. She rocked left and right, scooting one hip forward at a time until her feet touched the stool. Then she stood and wobbled down while I quickly spread towels and sterile drapes on the floor. With the light above us, I worked in the shadows, resting my knees and elbows on the floor waiting for the baby. My neck grew tired from looking up. Medical school had not prepared me for this.

Eleanor entered the room and stopped short. She walked to my side, stooped over with her hands resting on her knees. "Justine paid the thirty dollars and I put her to bed. I told you so." Having delivered what was on her mind, she took in the present situation. "What can I do to help?"

"Hold the table. It's starting to slide."

Lettie raised her body a few inches and dropped into a squat with her legs apart. She let out a groan, two deep breaths, a prolonged grunt, and a baby girl. Supporting the infant's head, I laid her on the drape-covered floor.

Drenched with sweat, Lettie pulled on the table leg and stood up.

"Now doc, that's the way to have a baby."

Dr. Buckner understood his patients lived by their own cultural beliefs that included superstitions, so standard approaches to treatment were neither practical nor effective. He practiced in terms his patients could understand. His positive outcomes would have impressed Mayo Clinic.

When I stopped by the office to pick up my $80 fees for the two babies I'd delivered earlier that week, Dr. Buckner stopped me from leaving. "You might want to see something they didn't teach us in medical school," he said, leading me in to a treatment room.

"Doc that old scary lady next door got mad at me over my dog and she put a hex on me. I hurt all over and I haven't slept in 3 days," the patient said, his legs dangling over the exam table.

"I'm going to burn that demon out of you with demon medicine," said Buckner, "but first I need you to lie down and stay real still."

He proceeded to rapidly inject twenty cc of calcium gluconate, double the standard dose, into the patient's vain in his elbow. Calcium gluconate, a classic safe drug used for muscle spasms and strains, had been around for many years, but its value was questionable. When administered in a vein, the medication needed to be injected very slowly, otherwise the patient would experience a sudden, warm flushing of the skin somewhere in the torso, lower abdomen, or rectal area.

The patient's eyes popped open wide. "Whoa! I feel it burnin' out that demon." He sat up, slid off the table and stood, his arms raised in celebration. "Hallelujah!" He strutted back and forth with his chest out and grinned. "Thank you, doc, thank you." Tears filled his eyes as he shook Buckner's hand and patted him on the back as the patient left his office. Buckner turned back to me.

"Thought you might want to see something they didn't teach us in medical school."

In another instance with one of Buckner's stubborn patient, a woman was experiencing an acute gallbladder attack. She needed to undergo surgery or risk complications and death. She had more faith in what she understood and declined surgery because of her fear of anesthesia and surgeons.

"I hear when they put you to sleep, they rape you or take a kidney," she said, defiantly resistant.

"I know the surgeon very well and he promises not to do that." Buckner patted her shoulder. "But to make sure of the problem, I have a recent invention that will tell me what it is. If the invention agrees with me, will you have the surgery?"

"Uh-huh," she said weakly.

"I'm going to step out to get it."

Slim electronic beepers that could be worn on a hip had recently entered the market. Buckner left the room and gave instructions to his nurse: "Wait thirty seconds before you page me and then slowly say 'gallbladder' three times."

Buckner reentered the room and unsnapped the beeper from his belt.

"I'm going to hold this magic machine over your belly and run it back and forth. It will tell me why you're sick and in pain." He waved the beeper inches above her exposed abdomen, slowly working his way down.

"Gallbladder, gallbladder, gallbladder," said an authoritative voice.

Buckner retold his unusual cases as matters of fact, never passing judgment on his patients or laughing behind their backs. He knew every patient's first and last names. Due to the limitations dictated by the culture in which he worked, his methods differed from the norm yet delivered good results. No government program matched the level of his care.

~~~

On a Monday, not long after I passed the six-month mark in primary care in Houston and had delivered eight babies, I received a surprise call from the Chairman of the Orthopedic Department of the Kansas City University of Medicine and Biosciences. A resident in the orthopedic training program had left suddenly for personal reasons. Without inquiring about my current circumstances, the chairman said the position was mine if I could report the following Monday.

I raced home. Tires squealed as the car braked to a stop in our Houston driveway. I bolted from the car and sprinted up the sidewalk onto the porch. "Mary!" I said, fumbling with the doorknob. I panted as I shoved aside the door and hurried through the living room. "Mary! We need to close up here and be in Kansas City by Monday."

"I'll start packing." I heard the smile in her voice, but she never even looked up from changing Lori's diaper.

I was committed to my decision, but I knew it meant dragging Mary and Lori across the country not knowing where we might land. Neither Mary nor I knew what to expect, and we avoided raising potentially painful questions. Amid preparations to leave the security of the known, I realized I held no confirming letter in my pocket. There had been no mention of income, not even a return phone number scribbled on a scrap of paper. I couldn't even recall the department chair's name. What if he changed his mind and someone else had already taken the position? What if Mary couldn't find a job?

By Thursday evening I had closed my practice, we made our farewells, and Mary had loaded a U-Haul with our belongings. At four o'clock Friday afternoon, we pulled out of Houston. I drove our 1964 Plymouth Valiant to which Mary had attached the U-Haul, and she followed with Lori in our VW Bug.

At two o'clock Saturday morning, we pulled into Mary's mother's driveway in Muskogee and headed to bed. Half an hour passed. I stared up at the ceiling.

"Mary," I whispered, "you awake?"

"Umm..."

"What do you think about getting up and going on—right now?"

"I've been lying here waiting to hear you say that." Once again, I could hear her smile.

CHAPTER 2

KANSAS CITY UNIVERSITY OF MEDICINE AND BIOSCIENCES

Kansas City, Missouri

1965-1968

On the first day of the residency program in Kansas City, I realized that Dr. Monaghan, Department Chairman and Chief of Orthopedics, was the opposite of Dr. Felmlee. Unlike Dr. Felmlee, who had made students feel comfortable by introducing them to new surroundings and procedures, Monaghan provided no orientation or warm introductions. The constant disdain in his voice made me feel I was in the wrong place at the wrong time, doing the wrong thing. Even when I stood next to him, he talked with others as if I was not present; Dr. Felmlee would have introduced me and included me in the conversation. Other staff members, however, accepted my presence and treated me respectfully as the new orthopedic resident.

Based on the brief and awkward meeting, I concluded the next four years of training would be a long four years. Maybe I could hold my breath that long.

On the second day, I wondered about the other two orthopedic residents who were supposed to be in the program. I soon learned the hospital had been approved for three, but the current budget allowed for only one, with the plan of adding another resident each of the next two years. Until then I was expected to cover the duties of three residents, including being on call 24/7 except for the fifth Sunday of a month, which occurred only three or four times a year. However, if an educational conference conflicted with that weekend, I was expected to attend. My duties included sitting through monthly department dinner meetings without a voice or vote. Meetings were held in rooms at restaurants and the subjects usually covered policy, equipment, and budgets.

The second week, Monaghan confronted me as soon as I saw him. "Why didn't you have the dressing changed on Reynolds in 211?"

"I was in the ER taking care of a fractured radius and ulna, plus a kid who'd stepped on a needle."

My defense didn't matter. Regardless of the credibility of my answers, he exhibited minimal tolerance. Sometimes he referred to a prior resident's cleverness or ability, implying I was being compared and didn't measure up. I immediately disliked the peers I had never met. Throughout a routine surgery, he continually criticized me. Either I didn't turn a screw into the bone fast enough or I screwed it in too fast. After he tied a knot in a suture, I wanted to ask if he would prefer I cut the ends too long or too short.

Quitting was not an option because I was responsible for the future of my family and I had no safety net. I wondered what kind of world I had entered.

During my second month, I accompanied one of my attending surgeons to an old two-story house turned hospital. With an anesthesiologist administering ether, I assisted with surgery to apply a plate in an elderly woman's fractured hip. The surgery room was on the second floor, and the building had no elevator.

"I'll call the city fire department. They have a stretcher with straps on it, and ours don't," the nurse explained. "It's hard to keep a patient on our stretcher and go down the stairs." She continued to write on the chart as she talked. "And if those strong guys at the fire department aren't busy, they carry our patients down for us. It's kind of a public service."

As luck would have it, the fire department was having a fundraising drive and the strong guys would be delayed two hours. With the patient still under general anesthesia, the scrub nurse and I lifted her under her arms from behind and the surgeon carefully lifted her legs. We carried her down a narrow flight of stairs, grateful for the depth of her slumber from the anesthesia.

I never had the occasion to return to that hospital, and thankfully, it closed within the year. By the 1960s most of these makeshift hospitals had closed because of increasing health and safety regulations.

~~~

The telephone rang at two o'clock in the morning. Mary groaned next to me in her sleep.

A patient had entered the ER with an injured hip sustained in a head-on collision. I was on call with no backup support while all three attending surgeons were out of town at a required medical seminar. At that hour, the ER was twenty minutes away—if I broke speed records.

I was completing my fourth month.

"What do his x-rays show?" I asked, rushing into the room.

Maxine, a nurse with years of ER experience, had seen hundreds of broken bones on x-rays. "I don't see a fracture but something doesn't look right. The femoral head doesn't match the socket."

The 31-year-old man writhing in pain lay strapped on a gurney. His right leg was half an inch shorter than his left. X-rays showed posterior dislocation—his right hip was out of joint.

He had been sitting on the passenger side of a vehicle when the collision drove both knees into the dashboard, forcing the ball of his hip up and over the back rim of the socket. The strong one-fourth-inch-thick capsule, which would not show on x-ray, had to have a large tear. I knew enough to recognize an emergency.

I broke into a sweat, my shirt sticking to my back, and I felt faint. Trying to hide my developing panic, I eased into a chair as though deep in thought. I had never seen a posterior hip dislocation, but I'd heard the term. I needed help. I phoned Mary and directed her to the textbook *Fractures and Joint Injuries* by Reginald Watson-Jones, published in 1941.

"Look at the index in the back," I said, checking my watch and making note of elapsed time. "Look up dislocation, then hip, then posterior."

"Found it."

"Read to me," I said, nervously tapping my foot.

Timing was critical. With the ball of the hip joint driven up and over the socket, life-giving blood to the ball had been choked off. Death rate of the ball was directly proportional to time dislocated. It could be measured in hours. Surgery was not indicated before an attempt was made to move the ball back into its socket.

With no anesthesiologist on hand, I needed to inject enough Demerol in the patient's IV to provide relief without causing an overdose. The only method of measuring enough Demerol was through pulse, respirations, and blood pressure measurement, which Maxine monitored. I walked a fine line between administering enough drug to relieve muscle spasms while preventing a fatal overdose. I knew the method to be crude. If I pulled on his hip before the narcotic produced its maximum effect, I would be tempted to administer more narcotic when the patient screamed in pain. I waited. His thrashing and yelling confused my decision-making process. Finally, his respirations and pulse slowed. My pulse was likely twice as fast as his.

I heard enough from Mary's reading to realize I needed an assistant in addition to Maxine. There was no one available but Maxine and me.

"I'm going to stand on a chair next to the patient on the gurney and Maxine will hold the desk phone to my ear."

"Okay," Mary said, believing in me before I dared believe in myself.

The textbook called for me to hold his knee and hip at right angles as if he were sitting upright in a chair instead of lying down. I needed to reverse the forces that drove his right hip backwards up and over the rim through the capsule of the joint. I locked the wheels on the gurney, stepped up on a chair with my right leg, and while standing over him, pressed my left knee into his pelvis.

"Flex the knee and hip to ninety degrees, which will help relax the muscles," Mary read.

"Okay." I bent closer to the phone while holding his leg.

"Apply steady traction holding the knee at right angles while the pelvis is stabilized."

With my body weight pressing his pelvis into the thin mattress, I held him stabilized like a wrestler in a ring and slowly pulled his leg with both arms until I fatigued. The patient groaned and cursed. He would have flown off the gurney had he not been strapped in.

"What does the book say now?"

"Repeated unsuccessful, painful attempts may cause muscles to go into spasm making reduction impossible."

I needed to rest. Maxine handed me the phone as she stepped onto the chair and steadied his knee in the air. I sat on another chair, elbows resting on knees. "Read some more," I said to Mary.

"If straight traction is unsuccessful with the knee flexed while steady traction is applied, move the knee toward the centerline. If the dislocation is not reduced within the first two attempts, further pulling increases the likelihood of fracture through the neck of the femur. Apply no more than two attempts."

Again, I stepped up on the chair, hovered over him, and transferred his leg from Maxine to me. Taking a deep breath, I pulled progressively harder as I held down his pelvis with my left knee. Maxine continued holding the phone to my ear.

"While traction is applied, rock and rotate the femur."

When I did, I felt a palpable "clunk." The patient's left leg lurched forward about an inch. I had pulled the ball from behind the socket and over the rim, seating it back into the socket. X-rays confirmed the ball was in place again.

"Success!" I told Mary. "Thanks for your help. You can go back to sleep now."

The patient ceased moaning and fell into a deep Demerol slumber. I flopped down on a gurney next to him.

~~~

By the sixth month of the residency I had learned to sit through long meetings with no opinion or input. Monaghan was engaged in a heated,

17

budget argument with Dr. Stepanek that was escalating. In his agitation, my chief's jowls shook like Richard Nixon's. I expected Monaghan to shake his fist, throw a shoe, or punch Dr. Stepanek, who sat directly across from him.

I waited, embarrassed, my head down. When the meeting came to an end, we filed out together and weaved between tables to the front door.

"Hey, Norris," Monaghan said, "let's stop at the bar. I'll buy you a beer."

Stepanek stopped and stared at him. "Why in the world would you want to do that?"

"I'm not mad at you." My chief's voice was surprisingly civil. "I didn't like the position you took, but I like you." He paused as though he were waiting to make a point. "You've got to be able to separate issues and personalities."

Within the hour, I found myself sitting at a sports' bar as the two professionals laughed and dissected the Kansas City Chief's last game. That night I'd sat with nothing to say and learned one of life's lessons in the process.

During a late lunch at Romano's cafe the following Thursday, Monaghan sipped his beer and elaborated on separating issues and personalities. The concept was a revelation to me. Ever since high school, if someone had made me uncomfortable I found myself disliking that person. I didn't know there was another option. My mentor supplied me with a tool that proved useful for the rest of my life.

That night when I arrived home, I found Mary waiting up, reading in bed.

"How are you and Monaghan getting along?"

I shrugged as if I had it all figured out. "I'm learning the system. Read up on upcoming procedures, don't ask questions, and be certain of my answers."

She nodded and smiled knowingly. I was once again reminded she could see through the best façade of bravado I could muster, but she respected me enough not to point it out.

I was grateful Monaghan didn't have the gift of perception my Mary did.

~~~

Monaghan began addressing me as if I was there to stay. He loaded me with additional responsibilities and reading assignments. For the first time, he asked about my family. When he was assigned as my attending physician, I was expected to follow him everywhere but the bathroom. I became aware of two personalities: In surgery, he was curt and frequently rude to the surgical crew; outside the hospital, he was a friendly man.

"I'll pick you up at the Kroger parking lot and we'll drive together," he said one afternoon. "Bring the current monthly *Journal of Bone and Joint Surgery*. You'll read to both of us. We can knock off a couple of articles each way." Because we worked out of two hospitals and drove the same route, I realized driving together was practical.

Five days a week I parked my car and stood in front of the Kroger supermarket at 7:00 a.m. waiting for Monaghan to pick me up. On the thirty-minute trips to and from the hospital, I read the journal aloud in the car. He drove a new Mercury that included the newly fabricated safety seat belts. Consistent with societal patterns, youth adapted quicker to change than older generations. I wore my safety belt, but he didn't buckle his, even though he earned some of his living from those who declined to do so.

We made the most of our daily trips together; he drove, I read aloud. But our education did not halt when we entered the hospital parking lot. The friendly attendant took it upon himself to provide us with the morning news as he took the keys. "The Snyder family is waiting on you to take Mama home. Crawford in 308 had a rough night. Leon in 314 hasn't had a bowel movement in three days, but the swelling in his foot has gone down." And so went the first year of my new program.

~~~

"Think of someone who is a good listener," Monaghan said as we sat down on a Thursday afternoon.

"My best friend back home."

"Name another."

"Mary."

"Does a poor listener come to mind?"

"Many."

"A good listener doesn't interrupt except to ask questions and drive the speaker deeper. I'm not a good listener. I want to jump in with my opinion," he said looking down at the menu, "but I'm working on it. There are three kinds of conversationalists: those who talk about ideas, those who talk about things, and those who gossip about other people." He placed his order for a meatball sandwich. "I try to keep our conversation about ideas, but sometimes I slip into gossip. If someone tells a story and begins, 'he said, then I said, then he said,' I want to doze off."

We sipped our beers.

Monaghan loved to talk orthopedics like sports fans talked sports. If Kansas City would have had an orthopedics bar, that's where we would have eaten our late lunches on Thursdays instead of at Romano's. His enthusiasm was my bonus. Although I had been programmed since first arriving in Kansas City to think of a residency as years to be endured, I began experiencing gratitude when orthopedic history, critical thinking strategies, and a successful surgery combined to change a life or limb.

Sometimes we sat in a booth and sometimes in chairs. I always followed his lead. A booth meant our subject for the afternoon was not serious. If it was serious and he was interested in what I was thinking, we sat in chairs so he could pull closer and lean in when making a point. To provide me with visualization of an instrument or prove a medical point, he often needed to sketch diagrams. He asked for a pen and paper from the owner with such frequency that Romano's began keeping a spiral notebook and pen for his use.

As I read in the car and we learned together, sometimes he'd say, "I don't know" or "I don't understand." I'd back up and read it again. I learned to respect him for his honesty. He began accepting me, not as a peer, but as his charge to teach. His brief answers expanded into deeper explanations as he methodically indoctrinated me with the history of why we were performing a given surgery. I learned most instruments and procedures were born out of necessity during a war. He could trace their evolution from the Civil War through the Korean War. While I listened that day, the U.S. was slogging through war in Vietnam.

He continued giving me orthopedic reading assignments throughout my residency, but as he became more comfortable with me, he included ethics, professional politics, personal development, and worldviews from a broader perspective. My limited background made me ripe for new ideas. He played on my curiosity and used me as an excuse to extend late lunches into long afternoon discussions.

After one Thursday lunch, I had stepped outside Romano's to reduce background noise as I listened to the long recording on my pager. Pagers of the era produced a loop recording containing a mixture of information. The hospital subscribed to a service that issued a three-digit identity number. Every thirty minutes, I turned it on and held it to my ear. A recording went something like this: "647 pick up a load of freight at dock C-3; 211 call home; 526 call the hospital." If my number came up with a message, I had to find a pay phone, so I always carried dimes to make two calls: one to notify the service company to delete my message and one to whomever wanted me.

A man who appeared to be drunk stopped but didn't interrupt me at first, just stared at me. "What's the score of the game?"

"I can't tell," I said, handing him the pager. "See if you can get it."

He held the pager to his ear, listening and stumbling back and forth. "Damnedest game I ever heard. Can't figure it out."

He pulled the pager from his ear, rolled it over in his hands, and listened with his other ear. Handing it back to me, he shrugged and wandered off down the sidewalk, shaking his head.

~~~

During my second year we had removed one of the earliest hip prostheses ever made. It had been inserted in a lady for a fracture of the head of the femur. We removed the metal ball because it was loose and any movement was painful. Monaghan replaced it with a tight fitting one. According to the family of the then 90-year-old, that prosthetic

21

head had been in place since the mid-1920s. Implants removed from patients are typically recorded, then discarded.

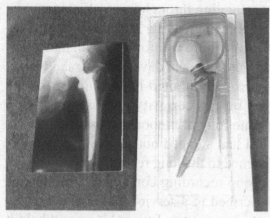

An Implanted Prosthesis and a Hip (Femur)
Prosthesis in Package

"Can I have the prosthesis?" I asked.

"What are you going to do with it? Start a collection of body parts?"

I ignored Monaghan's flippancy. The hip prosthesis became the first of many I removed and saved from patients during my career: rods, pins, screws, plates, and assorted orthopedic devices. Once rinsed and dried, my prizes returned to their bright, smooth metal-surface selves. A few implants and instruments came from shelves of outdated orthopedic supplies.

I eventually filled three large drawers and had a cabinet-maker build a large display case for my collection, all arranged in chronological order of introduction. Modifications and improvements through the years were also displayed. Some ideas lasted a decade or two before being replaced by innovations supported by evidence-based studies.

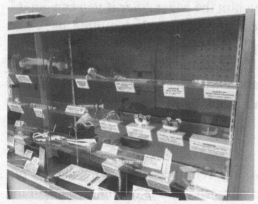

Display Case with Orhopedic Implants.
Some with Original Packaging and Others
Removed Over 40 Years

~~~

"You weren't the first on our list." Monaghan said as he sat directly across from me in Romano's one Thursday and gazed down at the table, too uncomfortable to look at me.

"What list?"

"The resident application list of those who had interviewed."

"What about it?"

"Before I called you two years ago, I called another guy. When our orthopedic resident left in a hurry for personal reasons, we needed a replacement right away." He paused, and I sensed he was baiting me.

"If you remember, I asked you if you could be here in one week, even though you lived in Houston." I nodded. "Well, the guy on my first call said his wife was working and he had two kids in school. He couldn't come for two months. So, I called the second on the list—you. If you hadn't answered or couldn't make it here in a week, I was going to keep going down my list."

I sat stunned, absorbing this new information. Why did he tell me? What was his motivation? I didn't understand why he'd told me now that it no longer mattered, and the knowledge hurt me deeply. The new information ranked up there with telling me I was a second choice in a marriage.

Whatever else we talked about that afternoon didn't register, and I drove home in a distracted trance. My hands began to sweat on the steering wheel, and I pulled into a roadside park. I realized that with a flip of the coin, my life would have changed forever if I had missed his call. I wondered what else had I taken for granted: My health? Healthy children? Was another coin of chance being tossed somewhere else in my life at that very moment?

Where might I be living and what might be the nature of my practice if I hadn't gone into orthopedic surgery? I understood that I'd been chosen from a list of eligible and competitive applicants from across the U.S. including two highly qualified former classmates who had applied for a residency slot. My acceptance into the training program had left me a bit cocky and comfortable with myself. With this new information I realized I was chosen because of luck, not because of my ability.

Just as abruptly as the shocking news from Monaghan had jolted me, I suddenly realized I could change my own destiny. I would apply my persistence to *earn* my luck. The new knowledge awakened thoughts that resolved me to learn life's rules: academic, social, and familial.

~~~

Occasionally one of Dr. Monaghan's partners joined us for lunch. On one occasion Dr. Bolin shared an afternoon with us at the café, along with Dr. Heim, a urologist. A bit of politics combined with some armchair quarterbacking for the Kansas City Chiefs made for lively conversation that grew more animated following the second round of beer. They began discussing their skills relative to those of their peers.

"You know how good each of us thinks we are?" said Dr. Heim. "Well, I may not know who the best urologist is, but I am very good at what I do. In fact, I don't want anyone operating on me except me."

"How does that work?" said Dr. Bolin.

"Look at it this way," said Dr. Heim. "Where on your body could you do your own surgery using both hands without a mirror?" Before we could respond he butted in. "With no assistant."

"Maybe the tops of my thighs," Dr. Monaghan said, "or something simple on the inside of my ankles, but I couldn't keep my legs crossed long enough. I have problems trimming my own toenails."

Dr. Heim puffed up his chest. "I did my own vasectomy."

I flinched, Dr. Monaghan leaned back from the table, and Dr. Bolin scooted back his chair. No one spoke.

Following a prolonged silence Dr. Monaghan raised his hand to the waitress. "This table needs another round of beers."

"I can do a vasectomy in fifteen minutes," said Dr. Heim. "Mine took a little longer because I was working upside down.

As the shock passed, we leaned forward, one by one.

"I turned forty last year and have four kids. That's enough. The kids and wife were out for Friday evening and I did the deed. The most comfortable spot was sitting on the toilet stool. I dragged a chair in front to hold the sterile instruments I'd brought from my office. If I bled, the blood would drip straight down." He did an eye sweep confirming he had our attention. "I had a shot of rum and Coke, then injected local anesthetic with a little bitty needle. It was a lot more sensitive than I thought so at that point I just drank straight out of the bottle. It took me twenty minutes and three stitches. And I can tell you, I walked mighty slow for the next few days."

"Did you miss any work?" said Dr. Monaghan.

Dr. Heim shook his head. "No. I went to work Monday. Climbing up steps was slow and taking a step down jarred me. I walked a bit straddle-legged." He did another eye drag around the table as though he was testing our belief. "When I was full of rum I thought some day I could circumcise myself. The next day I thought better."

~~~

Monaghan leaned on his elbows and locked eyes with me. "When I started practice in the 1950s, only M.D. orthopedic surgeons were allowed in salesmen's courses. I told a salesman I would use his products if he would let me wear his nametag to get in and sit through lectures. Courses were few, but I attended all possible. You've got to understand education means more to me than to most. Education denied is freedom denied."

He allowed me moments to process his last statement before he spoke again.

"That's the reason I have you read aloud in the car. That's dead time when we can learn."

He leaned back in his chair and nibbled on a potato chip.

"Times have changed and now any doctor can attend by paying the course fee. The sponsors want the fee and exposure. During your residency with us, the orthopedic department will pay your registration fee for any course available, and I'm sure the other three orthopedic surgeons will agree. I will pay for all other expenses, like travel and food."

"Who pays you to spend time to teach?" I asked.

"No one. I see it as my responsibility. When I was a resident, the chief of the orthopedic department was the designated trainer, but he never gave me a reading assignment or lecture. It was all 'because I said so.' I learn by reading, taking courses, and discussing cases."

Monaghan scooted his chair further in and leaned forward. "I see it as my responsibility to teach because he didn't."

Armed with this new information, I made a quantum leap of appreciation for education, especially orthopedics. Monaghan's frankness had also provided me with insight into his demanding character. I looked forward to reading together in his car the next day, making a transition from needing to learn to wanting to learn. I began attending as many additional courses as possible.

Every year orthopedic residents were required to take a written examination administered from our national office to document progressive education to meet the standards.

Monaghan carried the reputation of his residents scoring well.

I understood I was standing on shoulders of those who came before me even though I would never shake their hands or know their names. For the first time, I experienced the thought of wanting to pay back to my profession and looked forward to doing so, pondering on my drive home how I might pay him back.

~

"Let's get one more round of beer," Monaghan said as we finished a late Thursday lunch.

"But our work's done. Mary will be expecting me."

"We're not done until I say we're done. I want to explain some options about the knee surgery we just finished. But first there is another trap you can fall into if not forewarned."

Another pattern emerged. If he was going to talk at length and include details, he took a long slow swallow of beer. If he was already into the subject, the sips were short. He took a long draw on his beer and I knew to settle in for another long session.

"Never argue with success," he said. "You will have patients tell you how their neighbor rubbed ground-up squirrel scrotum on her arthritic knee and cured her arthritis, or that an aunt ate a Vick's salve sandwich under a full moon for pneumonia." He chuckled. "Our parents made us do some of that stuff."

"We practice in an evidence-based profession," he said, gesturing toward the journal on the table. "You need to find the balance. Listen and let your patients know you value their opinions, but dismiss anecdotal stories. When I was in training, I did what my chief demanded because he said so, never with reference to published information."

As he talked on and on, I thought about Mary. I wondered what made Monaghan so insensitive to my needs and to hers. I understood he had been in the military, which could explain his loud demanding voice and the fact that my personal life was a non-issue to him. I had no idea if he had been harsh on previous orthopedic residents since I had never met or visited with any of them.

My interest grew thin as he talked, and my mind questioned what he was like at home.

The effects of Monaghan's Thursday afternoon dominion didn't sit well at my home, especially when I arrived late, reeking of beer.

"I can't help it, Honey, it's my job. I'm expected to stay and discuss cases."

I knew my response sounded lame, but I believed the discussions to be teaching me something I couldn't learn in the operating arena or in a classroom.

"Don't you talk during the day?"

"Yes." I tried to sound authoritative.

"Well, I don't like him. Lori needs to see her daddy."

~~~

I figured I had been accepted as a member of the fraternity when Monaghan began talking about painful episodes of his early experience in surgery. He'd trained in the early 1950s when instruments were crude by later standards.

With enthusiasm for history, he told me the customary way to treat a fractured femur was to apply a plate with screws or prescribe months of traction in bed. After WWII however, a few Germans soldiers who came to the U.S. were discovered to have long rods inside their femurs. Historically they healed and returned to battle faster than any American soldier. U.S. hospitals purchased the rods to improve the method of fracture care. The rods arrived without instructions.

Monaghan admitted he and a resident had once struggled to position a properly sedated obese lady on her side, propping pillows around her and using a generous amount of two-inch tape to hold her steady. Monaghan made a five-inch incision on the side of her thigh that exposed both ends of a fracture. Using a bone clamp, he exposed the top bone out of the wound. With the tip of the rod inserted in the canal, he began driving the rod up the femur with a hammer.

The plan was to drive the rod up through the fracture in the center of the bone until it exited at the top of the femur. It would travel through muscle and bulge under the skin of her lower buttocks. When the bulge became evident beneath the skin, the resident was to make a half-inch incision for the rod to exit. It would then be driven up further until the lower end of the rod became flush with the fracture in the thigh. Both ends of the fracture would then be brought together and the rod hammered across the fracture until a half-inch of threads protruded from the top of the femur.

"Tell me when you see the rod pushing under the skin," Monaghan said to the resident on the opposite side of the table.

"I don't see anything. Keep pounding."

He continued to drive the rod further up the femur, waiting for the bulge under the skin to appear on her buttocks. When the lower end of the rod rested flush with the fracture, there was nothing else to pound. Perplexed, both surgeons tried to determine how the rod could have disappeared. They did not realize the obese patient under the drapes had rolled slightly onto her back.

"Let's roll her forward and look for the rod," Monaghan said.

When they rolled her forward, the two-inch surgical mattress pad came with her. The rod had exited the skin higher in her buttocks than anticipated, driving it through the sterile drapes and impaling the standard surgical mattress pad on the table.

"We nailed her to the table," said the surprised resident.

Baffled, they pulled the mattress pad and drapes off the rod, wiped it repeatedly with alcohol, lined up both ends of the broken bone, and

hammered the rod back down across the fracture. Monaghan intention-
ally left a half-inch of threaded rod protruding from the top of the femur, but covered with muscle. If it needed to be removed after healing,
he could simply make a one-inch incision, thread on a slap-hammer for
extraction, and give it a couple of good licks.

After listening to his misadventure in surgery, I leaned across the table.
"Holy mackerel! How did she turn out?"

My chief smiled. "She healed like we had done a hundred cases."
He dropped his shoulders with an exaggerated sigh. "I've told only a
few folks about the case, but you need to know your history."

During the next Thursday's lunch session Monaghan asked, "How
do you think the shoulder reconstructive surgery went this morning?
Should the bone graft have been bigger?" He spoke in a casual voice
as though he questioned me after every surgery. I was taken aback
because I was conditioned to listen, understand and agree—not be
questioned as a peer. "Should I have anchored the bone graft with two
screws instead of one?"

Confused for an answer, I responded with a non-judgmental reply.
"We could have saved time if you had closed the shoulder incision
while I closed the bone graft incision on his hip,"

I waited for a reaction but there wasn't one, so I kept eating.

He picked the Budweiser label with his left thumbnail and began
talking about something in surgery. I appeared to be listening as I sank
into my own thoughts. I wanted meaning with my training. Sitting in
the presence of someone with a passion provided an entry into meaning.
I began to realize that my experiences were defining my identity—at
least my identity as a surgeon. But I was also a husband and a father. I
was finding it difficult to be the best in all my roles.

Monaghan continued eating without looking up or displaying any
emotion whatsoever.

In that split second I felt we had come to a precipice in my surgical
training and both of us had crossed successfully over the gorge below.

I looked at the man sitting across from me; Monaghan must have a soft side that would eventually emerge.

~~~

On one of my few weekends off, Monaghan invited me to go fishing in a local lake. His partner volunteered to be on call. With Mary's blessing, I decided to go. I hadn't fished with friends or my daddy since high school.

There were many vital fishing supplies to take along on the trip, and one of the most important was cold beer. It served two purposes. If the fishing was poor, we would need comfort, but if the fishing was good, we would need to celebrate.

Monaghan rented a sixteen-foot aluminum runabout with an eighteen-horse-power engine. It wasn't enough to pull a small skier, but it managed to putter two adults and a cooler of beer around a lake.

After half an hour, one beer, and one bass that didn't qualify as a keeper, he pulled out a pack of chewing tobacco.

"Goes with fishing," he said, motioning to the package. "My wife won't let me chew around the house. One reason I go fishing." I pretended not to notice and tugged on my straw hat to protect my face from the intense sun.

As our boat drifted into the cool shade of a tree, we swapped our lures for plastic worms, and I welcomed relief from the sun for my pale skin.

"We're down on things we're not up on. Don't bring up a subject everyone in the room can't share."

"Like what?"

"Don't talk about a trip that others can't take or subjects not everyone can afford. Others don't want to hear about how smart your children are or how happy you are when they don't feel the same. They'll end up not liking you, so any issue you want to address gets started with you in the hole." He reeled in some of his loose line. "Manage things but lead people. If you get a chance, take the Dale Carnegie course. I wish I had."

He chewed his wad slowly, never looking up to see if I was listening. The fish weren't biting, but he didn't seem to mind. "Don't sit at a lunch table with the 'aginners.' You know, the table of doctors who are against everything and never make a problem-solving statement."

We were having conversation at the highest level of intimacy we'd reached as colleagues, talking about ideas. And it was fun.

~~~

As the months in surgical training passed and being on call became a pattern of late-night interruptions, some nights I was too exhausted to even react, especially when fast asleep.

"Answer the telephone," Mary said from her side of the bed.

I picked up the receiver and rested it on my chest. With an exasperated sigh, she lifted the phone and held it to my ear.

"Say hello."

With eyes still closed, I mumbled, "Hello."

I must have fallen back asleep because Mary was standing over me with my trousers in hand, telling me to get out of bed and go to the hospital.

She understood I was the first responder, but that didn't make it right.

~~~

My orthopedic training demanded long hours, and I began to understand I was missing involvement with my girls during a critical time in their development. Beth, our second daughter, was still a baby but Lori was old enough to look forward to being tossed by me high in the air and squealing with delight. She needed exposure to her daddy and I yearned to hear her squeal. We needed to have pillow fights and wrestle on the floor. These interactions became my fix, a kind of sedative for the chaotic pace and exhaustive hours required in my residency training.

"It's okay, it's your job." Mary attempted to alleviate my frustration.

But it was not okay. I could hear it in her voice.

Fretting about complicated cases and lacking time to read and being with my family, I was plagued by insomnia. My responsibilities consumed sixty hours per week, but Mary never complained. We both understood the residency had a defined ending.

When I called from the hospital telling Mary I was headed home, she began priming the girls. "Daddy's coming, Daddy's on the way home," she said, clapping her hands to create an atmosphere of celebration. By the time I reached home, Lori was pumped to begin the games—anything. For years to come Mary continued the tradition of announcing that Daddy was coming home.

The tradition worked both ways. I became excited because she stimulated our children, and I learned I could not just walk in and sit down. Walking in the door became an event. Sometimes I entered grunting and squatting like a gorilla with my hands high and chasing after the girls. Once Mary helped the girls make a paper flag colored with crayons, and the girls began waving it before I could get out of my car. Whether she made the announcement for our girls or for my benefit, I didn't care because everyone won. Lori was so excited that Mary often had a problem getting her to bed, but it was our time to play. Cancelling a circus in mid-act would have been easy compared to getting a call back from the hospital.

Mary had a plan and worked the plan. I loved coming home.

When Mary was six, her father had left her and her three brothers. Because her mother moved from one job to another, staying one step ahead of the landlord, Mary attended ten schools by the fifth grade. She soldiered on, made excellent grades, and learned to make friends quickly. As a result, she could walk into a social setting in one evening and make three friends. Others referred to me as Mary's husband.

Although Mary and I never talked about it, I needed to come through the door representing a dependable father—a minor celebration. I was sensitive to being absent in our home on long days for many days at a time. In our early years, I wondered if I was repeating the appearance of another generation of male absence, but Mary never mentioned it.

Worry dominated my thoughts, including how I would make up the lost days, weeks, and months to my girls. Other residents in training offered little personal advice because they were following their own voices. Monaghan's influence covered medical and political issues but limited instruction on personal and family development. I needed a mentor. Even a thin booklet regarding fatherhood would have been welcomed.

Each day I was learning to be a doctor while compromising my roles as husband and father. Passing written tests determined if I comprehended the massive volume of medical information, but being a husband or father did not require testing. If I missed a surgical step in a medical procedure, I received immediate feedback. I was drilled and questioned, and I learned from my mistakes. However, being a father was a lifetime job that offered little feedback; I might not know my performance scores for decades. Yet every day offered me a tiny window of time to play, love, and get it right.

~~~

Over the years Mary and I gained a rhythm of sharing small spaces—like brushing our teeth in our single sink bathroom and taking turns spitting toothpaste. From experience, we weaved and bobbed around each other avoiding head bumps.

"I have occasionally wished you had been my daddy. But I married you instead," Mary said one night, still bent over the sink. I continued brushing my teeth longer than necessary. She wiped her mouth and walked away to care for our girls, but her statement lingered in my head. I had never been wished to be someone's daddy.

Insomnia worsened as I fretted about complicated cases, lacking time to read and reflect on cases, just as I lacked time to be with my family.

I envied Mary's ability to fall asleep quickly, almost before she could get both feet off the floor, and certainly before a lengthy conversation in the dark. Hearing her deep regular breaths magnified my inability to fall into even a shallow slumber.

Some sleepless nights I slipped from bed to explore the refrigerator after Mary was asleep. But that night I quietly turned left into the girls' room. With eyes acclimated to the dark, I could see both girls, Lori in a small single bed along one wall and Beth in her crib along the next wall. They slept head to head.

Watching Lori breathe and then Beth, I found myself counting and comparing their respiration rates. Beth's rate was about right for her age, two more per minute than Lori.

In the dark I grew satisfied to simply be in their presence as an observer, without any action, words, or touch. By twisting the shade on a night-light, I altered the shadows on each face. I pulled my stool closer and marveled first at Lori, then turned my head and rested my chin on Beth's crib rail. Careful not to touch either, I leaned over to smell their bodies. Both smelled fresh, wholesome, and full of life that would burst forth from them when the sun rose in the morning. Beth radiated the scent of a baby, which she would soon outgrow, just as a puppy loses its distinctive lovable odor. Come morning they would wake making more noise than a rooster, with Lori running around chairs and squealing as if on a sugar high before running back to Beth as she tried to crawl to her big sister.

I wanted to supply them with a bulletproof vest of innocence, stability and confidence. But stability ranked first. As strong and feisty as Mary was, I sometimes saw her cracks of vulnerability. On rare conversations Mary whispered her dreams of stability under her breath. "We're going to live here long enough to drive a nail and hang a picture."

Responsibility passed over me like a heavy night shadow. I needed reassurance and advice that I was not getting on Thursday afternoons. I had once read the measure of a man is how well he takes care of his children. My work was pulling me away from being the father I wanted to be in their lives.

Would my girls ever understand I was torn between being with them and caring for people in pain? I asked myself which demanded more energy, being a good father or doctor. Hovering over their beds in the dark, I discovered I never wanted to have to make a choice.

When my nose began to run, I daubed it with the bottom of Beth's blanket, cleared a lump in my throat, and wiped away my tears.

With Lori asleep on her side and Beth on her stomach, I rested a hand on each of my joys. Their rhythmic breathing transferred through my fingers; as I savored the moment, I felt myself relax and become sleepy. I stood, replaced my stool, and tiptoed down the hallway to slide next to Mary, where I spooned with her, my left arm around her waist holding her close.

They can count on me, I thought, as I fell in line with Mary's breathing. Lying in the dark, I envied Mary's rhythmic sleep breathing and recalled a recent social event we'd attended with Monaghan and his wife.

"You're not going to get a divorce from Harold for working late are you?" he asked, attempting an ill-timed, light-hearted joke.

"No," she said, "there'll never be a divorce in our family, but maybe a murder."

I smiled in the dark, gave Mary a light squeeze, and drifted off.

~~~

It surprised me one Thursday lunch when Monaghan brought up the very subject that had been keeping me awake at night. "I keep preaching what you need to learn but skipped over what is more important. Be a father first. Knowing orthopedics shows what you know right away. Being a good father will require delayed gratification. How good you do as a father won't show for years. You can't do both. No one has that much energy. Both can't exist at the same level."

Over the next weeks his unreasonable criticisms and demands began decreasing. One lunch session he told me without remorse that his trainer, Dr. Simmons, had been cruel and biased.

"One would think the man had never dealt with an infection or a fracture that didn't heal, and I believed him for the first two years. My chief was cruel and dogmatic, and he believed he was infallible. Listening to him boast," he said, "one would think every case turned out perfect."

Both of us knew that perfection was an unrealistic expectation in the orthopedic profession. We had experienced that firsthand.

~~~

Although I qualified as an adult at age twenty-eight and was learning to assume more responsibilities outside my family, my value system had not changed since I was fifteen. I had only accumulated more life experiences. What I deemed at an early age to be funny, wrong or unfair had not changed but had only become better defined. I felt inadequate in so many ways and wondered if others could tell.

"How's it going with Monaghan?" Mary asked during one of our rare dinners together.

"It's easier to work with the other surgeons, but I learn a lot from him."

Sipping my coffee, I thought about how it was really going. I'd never told Mary about Monaghan's comparing me with former residents that he'd trained, implying that I didn't measure up. Nor did I complain about his overly critical assessments of my performance that seemed to have no basis. There was no need to burden her just to make myself feel better.

~~~

During one of my regular rotations, I began to experience first-hand the complexities and uncertainties that occurred in orthopedics. A twenty-two-year-old male came into the ER with a fracture in the middle of his femur. The break was two inches above the narrowest part of the canal, making him an ideal candidate for an internal rod. I assisted Monaghan as he made a five-inch incision on the side of the patient's thigh, exposing both ends of the fracture. He manipulated a rod into the canal at the fracture sight and hammered the rod up the center toward the top of the femur.

As planned, when the rod reached the top of the femur it broke through the thin shell to the outside of the femur without causing problems. As the rod continued to be driven higher, it appeared beneath the skin over his mid buttock. I made a small incision for the rod to exit. We lined up the fractured ends of the bone in the thigh and began hammering the rod down and across the narrow part of the canal. We only managed to move it two inches across the fracture into an even narrower part of the canal.

With each blow, a palpable tension invaded the room. Everyone in the surgery room knew we could split the femur. The sharp-pitched *bam-bam-bam* of the mallet was a comfort. If the pitch suddenly turned flat, the femur had split. With ten inches of rod protruding from the back of his right buttock, our options were limited.

"We need to pull the rod out and apply a side plate and screws before we split the femur," Monaghan said. Rods came with an attachment that could be threaded onto the upper end for insertion or extraction purposes. I threaded the attachment onto the protruding end and he delivered three blows. Everyone watched in silence. The rod didn't budge. He struck three more tentative blows.

The rod attachment functioned as a slap hammer. Instead of swinging a hammer through the air in a conventional stroke, a three-pound weight that surged up and down did the work. Monaghan's repeated pounding broke off the half-inch of thread on the end extending out of his buttock, deepening the mire we were in.

He backed away from the table, crossed his arms, and looked at the young man lying on his side with a ten-inch rod extending out of his body.

"Call maintenance and get two vice-grip clamps. They will need to be scrubbed, sterilized, and delivered to the surgery suite."

We covered the incision with wet sterile towels and waited for the clamps. When they arrived, I clamped them onto the protruding rod and attacked them with the mallet. We took turns trying to drive out the impaled rod; instead, we destroyed both clamps. Perplexed, Monaghan stepped back and stared at the protruding rod, a miniature flagpole jutting out of the patient's buttock.

Our dilemma was not mentioned anywhere in orthopedic surgery textbooks. We asked a nurse to pull out *Campbell's Operative Orthopedics* to review this section again. It didn't cover any such complication. However, the book described the procedure steps in detail, even providing a photo of needed instruments, all displayed on a surgery table. Monaghan eyed the photo thoughtfully.

"That's it," he announced suddenly. "The photo of instruments on the table includes a hacksaw. I always wondered what the saw was for. Someone's had this problem before. Call to maintenance for a hacksaw!"

Guarding the surrounding muscles with moist towels, we trapped the metal filings as we cut off the rod one inch above the protrusion from the femur. We returned to the incision on the side of the thigh, extended it over the fracture, and applied a plate and eight screws along the edge of the rod.

Seating a screw in bone is not like tightening one into metal or wood as snugly as possible with a tool. Instead, seating a screw in bone requires a surgeon to use his two fingers, and the final twist consists only of the amount of power the surgeon can create using the thumb and index finger. Tightening more could generate excess pressure on bone between the threads and cause the bone at the pressure sight to die. We completed the surgery.

By the end of eight months, the fracture had healed enough to risk removing the rod.

Following scar lines, I made a one-inch incision over the patient's right buttock and dissected through muscles down to the rod that protruded from the top of his femur. Anticipating the procedure, Monaghan had purchased the two largest vice grip clamps available at a hardware store. He also was aware that the extreme pressure that living bone creates against a rod would cause bone to resorb, but not visibly or on x-rays. In the second surgery with the larger clamp, a bigger hammer, plus the release of pressure on the rod from the resorbed bone, the rod came out in three blows.

"Let's go drink a beer and tell each other how smart we are," Monaghan said as we exited the surgery suite. I was beginning to see another side of my mentor, or he was finally allowing me to see a side of him that had been there all along.

The patient continued to heal well with the plate and screws, but the x-ray of his right buttock showed a sprinkle of rod-filings from our previous hacksaw adventure. He would carry a harmless remnant the rest of his life.

~~~

"What does Mary say about the conferences we have here?" Monaghan asked one Thursday when it was growing late.

"She's working with it," I said, summoning up my ever-developing diplomacy.

One Thursday when our lunch hit the six o'clock mark, I put both palms on the table in front of me. "I need to go home." I was becoming confused as to whether Monaghan's Thursday lunches with me were motivated by my company, his love of teaching, or his avoidance of home.

Ignoring my wife's concerns, and my need to keep her happy, he continued, his own agenda taking precedence over mine. "One more point I want to cover, and I want your opinion. We'll need another beer." He motioned to the bartender with two fingers.

"Pick your words before talking. If necessary, rehearse to yourself. If you shoot from the hip, it'll sound like it. If someone starts a sentence with, 'They say…' don't believe anything that comes after. That person never questions hearsay and doesn't know the different between myth and information." He rolled the saltshaker between his right thumb and index finger. "If someone starts with 'Everybody knows,' they're talking from a weak position."

He stopped the rolling motion, his face now sober. "If you want someone to like you, pay attention to the person's kids. My wife likes you and Mary because you pay attention to our kids."

He continued looking at the shaker without making eye contact.

"Never bring up an issue to be voted on unless you already know the outcome. Isolate each voter ahead of time and explain the issue, then ask for input. Once a person understands your position and interjects his input, he is no longer neutral. You've got him in your corner."

With every point made, he leaned forward, making sure I'd heard him. "Know how the votes are going to fall ahead of time whether days, weeks or months. If you're voted down repeatedly in an open meeting, you lose credibility. Save your voice for important issues."

The waitress set the fresh beers in front of us.

"In our profession, many issues are about hidden jealousy and pettiness, seldom for the common good. If in doubt, always take the high ground, perceived or real. Help the newcomer on staff, especially if he's a competitor."

He stopped talking to write notes in a small notebook regarding issues he wanted to address, rereading his list and scratching off subjects he'd covered.

"I know what I said. What did you hear?"

"I heard anywhere I go there will be politics and I'd better learn the rules."

Monaghan's question wasn't a test of my listening skills, but an assessment of the clarity of his explanation. I learned to give honest, evidence-based responses or concise summaries. Later in my residency he confessed, "Because of your feedback, I'm learning to articulate and better explain my theories."

~~~

Although Monaghan tended to repeat himself at our Thursday lunches and retell the same stories, over the next few weeks Monaghan started to tell me stories I'd never heard, personal stories that didn't always paint surgeons in a positive light. After one year of residency, Monaghan had prepared for an upcoming surgery on a fractured tibia by reading the recommended steps in *Campbell's Operative Orthopedics*. As surgery began, he wanted to show his chief he was prepared. "Dr. Simmons, I read in Campbell's which steps to take."

Simmons laid down his scalpel and shouted, "Monaghan, stop reading those damn books! I'll teach you everything you need to know about orthopedics."

Monahan's expression told me he was no longer sitting with me at the table but had returned to that hurtful moment when a respected teacher humiliated him in front of other doctors and staff. I felt a sudden and unexpected surge of empathy towards him, but I said nothing.

That afternoon Monaghan related another story about his chief. Monaghan had assisted him in a case for a non-healing, post-operative incision on a female patient who had undergone back surgery a month earlier. The incision had continued to drain, despite antibiotics. Without the benefit of a standard office x-ray, he returned the patient to surgery for exploration.

The surgical scar was four inches long, but the draining hole was less than one-inch. His chief extended the incision one-half-inch on each end. Using his dominant right hand, he wiggled his index and middle fingers into the new incision to blindly explore for the cause of drainage. He pulled back his hand with a sponge tucked under his ring and little finger, and as though stifling a cough, touched his mask with his right hand.

"Oops," Simmons said. "I've contaminated my hand. I need a new glove." He turned on his stool, peeled off his glove, and dropped it in the surgery trash container. Wearing a fresh sterile glove, he probed the wound further.

"I found the problem," he then said and, with a little drama, held up the two unabsorbed sutures for everyone to see. Sometimes a suture doesn't absorb and causes irritation and drainage until it is removed.

"I was the only one to see what really happened," Monaghan said in a hushed tone. "I speculated he left a sponge in the incision during the first surgery that showed on his office x-ray when the patient returned, but he never mentioned taking an x-ray. No one knew but me and he never mentioned it." I could tell from his expression that telling the story was painful for Monaghan. Memory can do that to us, replaying stories in our heads that with time become a mirror for our own lives and behavior. I wondered if Monaghan was beginning to see shadows of his chief in his own teaching methods. "I'm needing another beer. How about you?"

Twisting an empty bottle in his hand, he looked at me and spoke in a rapid almost self-conscious voice. "I've never told anyone that story. I was too embarrassed for him. But it happened long ago and he's dead." He took a deep breath. "He lied to me."

We sat in silence.

Because I did not show indignation or pass judgment, he continued to tell me a story from the early 1950s. "Simmons had taken an elderly lady to surgery to repair a fractured hip. X-rays of the era were often blurred and multiple x-rays were taken before an acceptable one was developed. Portable machines were not yet available. Therefore, he performed the procedure in the x-ray department as opposed to the surgery suite. Opening the hip, he inserted the plate and screws. On completion, he took a final x-ray and discovered something he hadn't expected: he had pinned the wrong hip.

His chief then proceeded to pin the hip with the fracture. When he finished, he covered his error by telling the family he'd repaired the broken hip, but the x-rays of her good hip showed it was also very weak and could fracture at any time. Therefore, for the patient's benefit, he'd pinned it as a preventative measure."

"He never told me," Monaghan said, "if he charged for two procedures and I wasn't about to ask."

Although embarrassed for witnessing his trainer's error, Monaghan used the story to explain why he took such great measures to confirm he was indeed operating on the correct hip. During my four years, he probably told me the story three or four times, and it was what was on my mind as I encountered my own problems later in practice.

"I've told this story of the wrong hip to only a few, including my wife," he said.

I thought it reflected well on my training that he would tell me such personal stories. I was being spoon-fed and homeschooled—a blessing bestowed on only a few residents. I suspected he was using his story to rationalize his counterproductive approach with me.

Although he allowed me to perform entire surgeries in the final months, his criticisms continued. Undoubtedly, he would say it was a product of his training. But even though I had been exposed to the same treatment, I vowed to function differently in my own practice. If orthopedic residents were ever on my service, I would correct with positive reinforcements.

~~~

Throughout my residency Monaghan kept me off balance. The curt-talking man in surgery was not the one who sat across from me sipping a beer and eating a sandwich. In Romano's atmosphere, he was quick to laugh and eager to share learning experiences. Although I never knew what to expect, I was developing two personalities: one for surgery and one for Thursday conferences. "Conference" is the term he used when he called his wife, and I began doing the same.

~~~

In one surgery with Monaghan, I was assisting on a femur fractured into four pieces. "How do you know which bones to line up first?" I asked.

"You get the assembly of pieces out of order enough times like I have and you get the hang of it," Monaghan said with a brush-off answer. He responded as though his answer was a joke, but I heard the operative word: experience. Surgeons are forced to make quick critical decisions based on the intangibles of experience and intuition. Despite the best of intention and skill, mistakes are made and their results may be permanent. Experience exposed me to ways of learning from my mistakes. If I made the incision a bit low, I found myself struggling to see the problem and required another five minutes. The next time I made an incision, experience told me to make the incision two millimeters higher. Each case thereafter became easier. Expertise is the art of decision-making and comes from experience. However, the tuition can be high.

THE LIFE
OF A SURGEON

1968-2010

A BRIEF HISTORY OF ORTHOPEDIC SURGERY

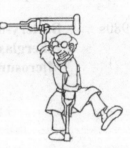

Rags and Sticks
Hammers and Hacksaws[1]
Opium, Ether, Chloroform, Morphine
Plaster of Paris Casts

1890s   **Sterilization** by boiling or steam
           First Hip Replacement using ivory for femoral heads
           X-rays[2] discovered
           Internal Fixation with hardware-quality plates and screws

1940s   **Rods and Pins** down center of hollow bones
           Power Saws and Drills

1950s   **First Generation Fluoroscope** to provide multiple x-ray
                 views during surgery

1960s   **Total Hip Replacement** plastic cup, metal ball, and dental
                 bone cement
           External Fixation with rods and pins[3]

---

[1]   Still in use from hospital maintenance departments when necessary.

[2]   Considered the first major advancement in orthopedics because bones could be set without surgery.

[3]   Pain free and effective.

1970s **Total Joint Replacement**[4]
Plastic Bones for practice before surgery
Arthroscopy[5]
Compressed-air Drills and Saws

1980s **Battery-operated Drills and Saws**
Fiberglass Casts
Microsurgical Instruments for reattaching extremities

---

[4] Considered the greatest advancement in all of medicine for pain relief.

[5] Most commonly performed orthopedic practice.

CHAPTER 3

ORTHOPEDIC PRACTICE

Tulsa, Oklahoma

1968-1974

When I considered locations for an orthopedic practice in the late 1960s, it was important to consider the ratio of doctors and their fields of practice to a city's population. As a rule of thumb, a primary care doctor needed a base population of 1,000. Thirty primary care doctors were needed to fill a two-hundred-bed hospital, supporting five internal medicine physicians and one general surgeon. A town with less than 25,000 could not support an orthopedic surgeon.

Orthopedic surgery of the time required large incisions on backs, legs, or arms. Fractures and trauma could easily constitute half an orthopedic practice. The introduction of total joint replacement gave the surgeon more tools and improved options. Arthroscopy, CAT scans, and MRIs enabled them to see problems hidden deep within arms, legs, and backs, allowing for plans to be developed long before an incision was made. Care of fractures and trauma decreased as a percentage of an orthopedic practice. We were doing more with smaller incisions, many only the size of a hole for a button. A surgeon could offer more services to fewer people. Within two decades a community of 15,000 and a city hospital could attract and support him.

I joined a practice with two seasoned orthopedic surgeons in Tulsa, Dr. Campion and Dr. Peele, gentlemen who daily expressed their support. I learned new techniques, shaved valuable time from procedures, and picked up effective skills for managing the office—information that would have taken years to learn on my own.

Campion understood and practiced the art of both listening and talking with patients, making them feel special. One such patient he cared for over the years needed to have an appendectomy. She was very sick and ran the risk of complications if her appendix was not removed soon. Although an orthopedic surgeon would have no reason to be present during her abdominal surgery, she refused to undergo general anesthesia unless he was present. The request was not rational, but she wouldn't compromise, so Campion gowned up and held her hand until she was under anesthesia.

When my parents visited Mary and me in Tulsa, I gave them the tour of our orthopedic facility. "This is what we talked about the summer I graduated from high school," I told my father, nodding toward my new office with my name on the door.

"What are you talking about?" my father said.

"Way back then you asked me why I wanted to go to college and I couldn't give you a good answer. Well, my answer is this office and my work. I have purpose."

My mother grinned.

~~~

In the early months of my practice in Tulsa, I found myself opening my mouth and hearing Monaghan. His shadow remained ever-present, looking over my shoulder to confirm I was practicing what I'd been taught. If I had questions when I was on my own, I took comfort in knowing I could retreat into our cocoon at Romano's for the answer. The history of every instrument I picked up passed through my mind, including the importance of its evolution explained to my by Monaghan. Silent embarrassment engulfed me as I reflected on my lack of appreciation for his efforts.

My responsibility resided in passing along his philosophy. I gave myself permission to modify or expand his understanding of an academic or social issue. When a complex case entered my office, I retreated to his evidence-based answers.

After two years in practice, his influence mellowed me enough to write him a two-page letter to thank him for not only teaching me to be a surgeon, but for introducing me to a bigger world. His life lessons taught me the importance of picking my battles carefully and maintaining restraint for those not worth the effort. So when I found myself sitting in mundane meetings with an urge to make my opinions known, I listened instead to his voice in my head, telling me to be still: If I have an opinion on every issue, I have influence on none.

Whenever I met Monaghan at conventions he hugged me shoulder to shoulder in public long before it became fashionable for men to show such affection.

"Let's skip that next lecture and go to the bar," he said. "I'm buying. I don't want anyone joining us because we are going to have a long conversation, just like at Romano's."

I nodded and pulled out a chair at a table.

"Let's go to a booth. It's more private."

As if I were still in training, I followed him to a booth.

"How are Mary and the kids? How's your practice? How are your partners?"

Although he was curious about my wellbeing, he still controlled the conversation, but the tone was different. He genuinely cared. His words were more selective and less dogmatic. I sat across from a different man.

～～～

During the 1970s, board certification for orthopedic surgery involved two stages. Following a minimum of two years in practice, and if the applicant passed the written and oral examinations, six months later the applicant underwent an on-site medical records inspection by two experienced examiners and an observation of a surgical procedure. Most failures to pass occurred due to the medical records inspection.

Failures were not usually from surgical ability but from lack of medical documentation regarding justification of surgery.

A quality hospital chart needed to reflect the original decision-making process justified by independent evidence, such as laboratory and x-ray reports. Since chart documentation was such a routine part of practice, minor poor habits were easily overlooked in a busy practice, which is why the medical records inspection was often the culprit for failure.

I was eager to begin the long certification process.

A surprise call came from Monaghan. "How about me flying down and doing a courtesy chart examination? It is unusual, but legal. Be glad to supply a practice run on your charts." He cleared his throat. "I can fly down some morning, examine your charts, and fly back the same afternoon." I was still thinking about it when he continued, "I would like to do that for you. If we finish in time, we could visit."

Over lunch on the day of the complimentary examination, he proposed an idea. "If you've got time some Friday night, I'll meet you at Joplin, halfway between Tulsa and Kansas City. We can spend the night having a leisurely dinner, drink a beer, and visit. No agenda."

As I listened to his suggestion, I realized that while my practice was consuming my time his was slowing down. Trying not to show my reluctance, I agreed on a date.

When I arrived in Joplin at our appointed meeting spot, Monaghan shook my hand and gave a courtesy side-to-side shoulder bump. He was upbeat and eager to visit, but my mind wrestled with issues back in Tulsa. During our long dinner, he revisited old events and exaggerated the past. I kept thinking about all the work waiting for me back home. I was glad to meet with him, but we couldn't recreate the world of Romano's. He'd been my constant teacher and I'd learned much about the subtle nuances of my profession from his stories and teaching, but he was no longer my teacher, he was my peer.

Within a few hours, he wanted to commit to a future date to meet, but I fabricated one lame excuse after another. We never met again outside of formal meeting and conventions. When we met at conventions, he always insisted on buying dinner. The adage, "It takes a long time to grow an old friend," kept running through my mind. He wanted to nurture the friendship with more social visits, but I rationalized I was too busy. I managed to delay seeing him between conventions until he died.

I am forever sorry.

Monaghan's influence continued decades after he left this world in 1998. His coaching provided a perspective of life and education. He helped me define values, understand my roots, and become the surgeon I am. When I talked with orthopedic residents in our program, I heard his voice coming from my mouth, but his words originated deeper than in my throat.

~~~

Working as a surgeon in private practice presented me with new challenges on a regular basis. Although each procedure that I completed successfully added to the treasury of surgeries I could perform, I didn't reach the confidence level in my career I had imagined for so many years during my internship: a time when a surgical procedure no longer felt daunting or challenging.

Two years into my practice, a patient presented with disabling pain from a bone spur and ruptured cervical disc in her neck. I had watched a surgical procedure in which a cervical disc had been removed and fused with a bone plug, but I hadn't even assisted in the procedure. I didn't want to perform the surgery myself, but I didn't have anywhere to send her, and she needed immediate relief. Her cries of pain convinced me to act regardless of my comfort level. Her ruptured disc needed to be removed because it was pinching a nerve. The bone spur also needed to be removed and followed up with a bone graft.

The surgery required an incision in the front of her neck, dissecting down through critical nerves and blood vessels until I reached the bone. In preparation, I had read, reread, and studied pictures in an anatomy book.

I took a deep breath and drilled a sixteenth-inch diameter wire from front to back between two vertebrae and shot a side-view x-ray to confirm I was at the correct level. I slipped a half-inch drill with a hole in the middle over the wire. When I had watched the one cervical surgery, the surgeon used an air-powered drill. The high-speed drill was beyond my experience. Instead I used a slow-turning, hand-driven drill to prevent over-drilling. The drill needed to be taken down to within one-eighth-inch of the spinal cord.

My pulse raced. I felt as out of place as student pilot on his first solo flight, flying the plane with his left hand while holding the training manual in his right. Monitoring the depth by taking serial x-rays from the side, I teased and lifted out the offending ruptured disc in small pieces that impinged the nerve. When I could determine the nerve rested without being pinched, I nibbled off nearby bone spurs with a side-biting instrument.

A bone graft from the donor site required a second incision on her pelvis. While I worked on her neck, the assistant prepped and draped the appropriate pelvic crest. I made an incision over the crest and lifted the muscles and nerves apart, exposing the top of her pelvis. Using a hollow drill, I harvested a core of bone exactly one half inch in diameter, the size of the hole between her cervical vertebrae. I returned to her neck, retracted the muscles, nerves and vessels and exposed the prepared hole.

Traction on her neck provided enough space between the cervical bones to gently tap the round bone-plug into the prepared hole. A nurse released the traction, and side-view x-rays confirmed good positioning of the new bone plug.

My heart did not slow until late that evening.

She obtained excellent relief from neck pain. As expected, however, she continued to have hip pain from the donor site for weeks.

~~~

In my experiences within the shared private practice, I came to appreciate that Dr. Campion never used medical jargon with patients and families. When he dictated, he said something along the lines of, "I performed a closed reduction of his left distal radius and ulna and the post reduction and casting x-rays showed satisfactory alignment in

both the AP and lateral views. A full arm cast was applied with immo-
bilization of his elbow at ninety degrees." However, when he visited
with the family, he explained, "I set both bones in your son's wrist, and
they'll grow strong and straight as six o'clock." Dr. Champion taught
me to explain enough to satisfy a patient and family, and then shut up.

As my awareness of communications evolved, I sometimes finished
an explanation with one of Monaghan's favorite lines: "I know what I
said, but what did you hear?" I tried to be diplomatic when doing so,
as I didn't want to embarrass anyone. Since a patient's expectation is
much different than a doctor's, I wanted to make sure I addressed them
early on, especially regarding x-rays. In general, the patient values an
x-ray as an absolute answer, but a doctor sees an x-ray only as supporting evidence.

~~~

Four years into my practice, a confused, elderly woman had fallen
out of bed in a nursing home, and the ambulance brought her to the hospital at four o'clock in the morning. The ER physician had examined
her, and in the x-ray found a fractured right hip. He ordered five pounds
of traction applied to her right leg to limit movement and relieve pain.

Six-thirty the following morning, I reviewed the x-rays of her right
hip in the radiology department, and went directly to the patient's room.
I introduced myself to two family members who had stayed the night.
They informed me their mother had been confused for months and
unable to communicate in the nursing home. The combined effects of
trauma, medication, and the patient's dementia meant I couldn't obtain
a medical history from her.

When I examined her, I explained to her family about fractured hips
in lay terms, as well as the need for surgery. I included her outcome was
guarded due to her age and general poor health. Explaining in greater
detail, I told them if we didn't stabilize the fracture with a pin and plate,
she would remain in pain and couldn't move from side to side or sit
up. The pain would also prevent her from sitting on a bedpan. In short
order, she would develop skin break-down with ulcers beginning with

pressure points, back, and buttocks. Within a week she would have probably develop pneumonia from lack of movement because of the pain. A urinary catheter would be required, followed by a high probability of a urinary tract infection. So stabilizing the fracture would enable the medical staff to prevent a predictable, slow, and painful death.

Following a pre-surgical evaluation of her heart and lungs by an internal medicine physician, she was cleared for surgery. Although she was a poor surgical risk, surgery was the best option. The internist advised me she was in the best health possible under the circumstances and waiting would not improve it. The window of optimal time was closing.

The staff rolled her into surgery on the same bed in which she had spent the night. Considering her age and complex medical history, general anesthesia wasn't the best option. Therefore, the anesthesiologist gave her a little sedation, then turned her to her side and administered a spinal anesthetic. Within minutes she was pain free.

I removed the fraction from her right leg and helped transfer her to the fracture table. Contrary to a flat surgical table that supports the entire patient, a fracture table is composed of segments and moveable arms. A patient's legs can then be manipulated into multiple positions and maintained while the surgeon does his work.

We positioned her to straddle a padded post with both feet strapped into footplates. By turning a crank, progressively controlled traction was then applied to line up the fracture pieces of her right hip. Since I couldn't see the alignment with the naked eye, I ordered x-rays of her right hip, even though it can be difficult to get an accurate image in this area of the body.

Sometimes the fracture could not be seen due to a combination of good alignment, poor bones from lying in bed, and general limited film quality. A repeat film would require the loss of valuable time under anesthesia and lengthen the surgery. Her poor health could not tolerate more time. We proceeded with scrubbing the site and draping for surgery.

Surgery has a subtle rhythm one acquires over the years: step one, step two, step three. . . . There is an intuitive sense of all being right with the world when the rhythm of the procedure falls into place.

As we continued to prep the patient, low professional chatter permeated the room. Instruments clinked. The low hum of fresh air passed through the filters. There was no sense of anything being amiss. But I could sense my rhythm was off and my intuition was active.

Picking up the scalpel, I laid the cutting edge against the skin and began an incision. I stopped at one inch. A tsunami of emotions, anxiety, fear, and apprehension, flooded me.

"Something's not right," I said without inflection.

Vague foreboding washed through me. Expectant eyes turned my direction. I walked to the x-rays. I could not see the fracture. Perhaps I had lined up the fracture too well to be seen.

"X-ray her other hip," I said.

We waited in silence for the x-ray technician to take a new x-ray of her opposite hip, leave the room, walk down the hall to the darkroom, develop the film, walk back down the hall to our room, and hang the results on the view-box. Everyone in the room could see the fracture of her left hip.

My heart rate made a vertical trajectory and I became nauseated. I slowly shook my head in disbelief. Because x-ray images do not indicate which side of the body is being shown, a left or right marker is always placed on the film by the tech before the x-ray is taken. In this case, the "right" marker had been used instead of the "left" marker the night before in the ER.

Monaghan's voice rang in my head. "When things go wrong in surgery," he told me one night at Romano's, "I fantasized I would faint and someone else would take over. And then when I awoke, the problem would be solved." We had both laughed. But in that moment of surgery, I had the same ridiculous fantasy.

I closed the small incision on her right side with two sutures and a small dressing. We removed the traction from her right leg, reassembled the fracture table, and placed her left leg in traction. Quality x-rays revealed the fracture in her left hip to be in good alignment. I proceeded to place a standard large fixation screw into her femoral head and neck, and anchored it to the side of her femur with a six-hole plate and screws. The rest of the surgery went well.

Stopping outside the door of the waiting room, I swallowed, inhaled a deep breath, and faced the family. I explained the sequence of events, including the small incision on her good side requiring two stitches. "I am responsible and can't blame anyone else. A 'right' marker was placed on her x-rays instead of a 'left.'"

I explained when the nurses and doctors saw the traction on her right leg we assumed it was the fractured side. Although the sequence of errors didn't start with me, I was the captain of the ship and responsible for all activities. Once she entered the operating room, she became more my responsibility and casting blame wouldn't help anyone.

Her daughter said, "Last night the doctor placed the traction on her right leg, and I wondered about that. But Mom was confused and didn't complain."

When I expressed genuine remorse, I think they felt sorry for me. They understood my pain and showed support. Her son shook my hand and his sister gave me three light pats on my back.

The patient healed well and eventually returned to the nursing home. Because I owned the responsibility, I ended with a good relationship with their family and cared for other members over the years.

~~~

Practicing as a orthopedic surgeon had its comical side that embellished daily life and acted as a balance for the serious work performed in the surgical arena. One such entertaining episode occurred during my early days in the Tulsa practice.

A couple of fellows had attended a University of Tulsa football game and had arrived early. They chose to sit in the end zone seats to gain a different perspective. TU was playing the Air Force Academy, and the visiting team had brought along their falcon mascot and pretty cheerleaders.

"Look at that falcon's claws. I'd hate for that black-eyed mother to get hold of me," one said as he peered through the binoculars. "But that second cheerleader from the left would be okay."

TU was practicing kicking field goals. A football sailed through the goal posts and struck the center of his binoculars. He never saw it coming.

"I woke up with people around me and blood everywhere," the young spectator told me the next day.

The binoculars punched a perfectly round laceration around each eye, but not deep enough to require sutures. Not visible, but more painful, the blow also created a whiplash injury when his head was violently thrown back. He had been admitted to the hospital for care of his whiplash.

The following morning, bruising began to appear. By the second day, he sported a perfectly symmetrical dark blue mask. Although the prognosis was good, he required pain and muscle-relaxing medication. He remained hospitalized for painful whiplash.

A makeup artist from Hollywood couldn't have painted on a better mask. My patient looked like Zorro peeking through his mask. He could look left and right, which was a bit scary, but very funny, even spooking the nurses because they felt like he was spying on them. Because of his whiplash injury, his neck pain kept him from turning his head—so he could only move his eyes. I had to stand at the foot of the bed for him to see me.

"He looks like one of those old movies, where a villain peeks through a portrait painting where the eyes have been cut out," said the head nurse. "He's watching our staff."

Each time before I entered the room, I had to take three deep breaths to keep from laughing at his mask and shifting eyes. Twice, I had to leave to regain my composure before finishing my visit.

"It's not funny until I scared myself looking in the mirror," he said, high on pain meds.

Two days later, he left the hospital and returned to my office the next week.

"You're not going to believe this," he said in a serious manner. "A policeman pulled me over for not coming to a complete stop at a sign. He walked up to me, and when I looked up, he backed off." He nodded eagerly as if to convince me. "That ain't all. My eyes are so scary my wife made me sleep by myself the first three nights after I got home. And my boss keeps me out of sight working in the mailroom."

With physical therapy, he made a slow but full recovery over three months. On his last appointment with me, only by looking closely could I see a small curved white scar below each eye.

~~~

The same time that the Nixon/Watergate investigation dominated the news, medical seminars and orthopedic journals revealed groundbreaking news of experimental total joint replacement. Those of us in practice hoped to learn to relieve painful arthritic joints.

A simple envelope in my mail contained a registration form to attend one of the first courses offered in the U.S. for total knee replacement. With the $100 registration fee and completed form, I drove straight to the post office and paid the extra $1.25 to send it airmail.

Surgeons with young faces, gray hair, and balding heads filled the one hundred fifty seats in the lecture hall. We learned the physics and theory behind the company's implants, but the speakers delivered only nonspecific verbal instructions, providing no printouts or diagrams on how to cut and prepare the bones to receive the new implants. An orthopedic surgical implant company sponsored the course.

"What special instruments are needed?" asked a surgeon after the presentation.

"We're working on that. We have a booth set up in the hall with some experimental instruments, but in the meantime, use whatever tools you have in your garage."

The three components of a total knee replacement were also for sale in an adjacent booth: metal surfaces for both sides of the knee and a high-density plastic for the kneecap. Hospitals and surgeons could buy all three parts, even though they would arrive without instructions.

Some surgeons attended class, returned home, and promptly performed their first total knee replacement. Other surgeons delayed for years, waiting to watch a case or two. I felt the price tag for not getting the surgery right the first time was too high. In the new field of total joint replacement, exacting bone cuts were land mines. Marginal errors could have been disastrous.

~~~

My senior by about 25 years, our hospital pathologist was quiet-mannered and approachable. He ate lunch earlier than most, so I arrived early. After returning home from the knee replacement conference, I waited for him to sit down at a table before I casually set my tray across from him, hoping to negotiate what I needed before anyone sat next to us. A friend who was an orthopedic sales representative had given me factory rejects for one knee replacement, but I needed help from the pathologist to proceed with my plan.

"Dr. Wasserman, I need a leg."

"What?"

"I'm going to perform my first total knee replacement and I need to practice on a leg. A whole leg."

"Never heard of such a thing."

"I haven't either, but I have to start somewhere. I can't do this without your help. No one would see the leg but me and we would be providing a future service to our hospital. I'll have it back in an hour. I have patients with crippled knees crying in pain and trying to survive day to day on narcotics."

I leaned forward and took advantage of his silence. "If you can't help me, I can't help them. If you can come up with a leg from the dead, I can relieve pain in a leg of the living."

The leg would come from a patient to be incinerated following an autopsy.

He looked around the room and back at me. "I'll see what I can do and let you know."

After lunch I approached the hospital maintenance supervisor. "I'd like to use that big bench vice in your shop to hold a leg."

"Okay. Something I can help you with?" he said before fully understanding the question.

I went on to explain what I needed to do, taking care to tell enough without upsetting him.

"Ahem." He drew in his chin. "Well…"

"I'll take that as a yes and let you know when I need your shop. After it closes, of course, and everyone has gone home. I'll clean up any mess. You'll help people suffering with knee pain."

I waited for a leg. A month passed before Wasserman stopped me in the hall.

I saved you a leg from the hip down," he whispered. "I have it in the refrigerator. Can you pick it up tomorrow?"

As if I were making an illegal drug purchase, I timed my trip to the autopsy room when no one was around. The leg was wrapped in a sheet. I carried it to the maintenance shop in the basement, well aware I carried a body part of someone who had lived and probably loved. I did not want to know the person's name or the circumstances of the death.

Only two people knew of my plans because I wanted to avoid any chaos in the shop and didn't want the hospital administrator to throw a net over me.

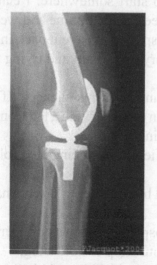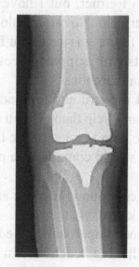

<table>
<tr><td>Side View of Total Knee
Replacement</td><td>Front View of Total Knee
Replacement</td></tr>
</table>

The next day, alone in the basement with the leg, I taped the foot to the workbench and bent the stiff knee several times with force to gain ninety degrees. After securing the head of the femur in the vice, I made a seven-inch incision along the side of the kneecap and inverted it to expose the entire joint, essentially turning the knee wrong side out.

Without cutting guides, I backed off and eyeballed the bone cuts. Using a reciprocating saw, I made my first cut. Satisfied with the angle, I was making my second cut when a guy sauntered into the maintenance shop behind me. Walking to one end of the workbench, he stopped and stared bug-eyed as he processed the scene. He vomited on the floor beside me before he could speak or turn around. Without missing a step, he hurried out the door, retching all the way.

The small errors I made on the borrowed leg enabled me to adjust my technique and successfully perform my first total knee replacement on a middle-aged woman one week later. With the cooperation of the hospital pathologist and shop supervisor, I could relieve disabling pain and improve the quality of life for my patients.

~~~

On one occasion in surgery, a salesman was present while I worked on a total knee replacement. After removing the appropriate amount of bone on the femur and tibia, I applied the temporary implants to size the joint. When I confirmed the size needed, I asked for a permanent left medium femoral component. The salesman stepped outside the surgery suite to retrieve it from his extensive inventory.

We waited unusually long for him to return.

"I'm so sorry," he said. "I don't have a medium femoral component in my hospital inventory and my office doesn't have the size you need."

The room fell so silent I could hear the patient breathing on the anesthetic machine. All eyes turned to me, waiting for my response. I recalled Monaghan saying, "If you have a crisis that is not time critical, don't do anything."

I considered removing more bone to adapt to a different size, but that choice was inappropriate for the patient's body proportions. I could not compromise. I became aware of the two residents waiting and watching, and unknowingly learning how to respond. I had the option to yell, curse, or blame someone.

Following a long, slow, deep breath, I said to the salesman, "Walter, where can you find a right medium total knee?"

He left the room and was gone less than three minutes.

"One is on its way from Oklahoma City," he said as he came back through the door. "With a highway patrolman going way over the speed limit, I can hand it to you in forty minutes."

I washed the incision with the power irrigator and covered it with wet towels. We waited and waited in the silent surgery suite. Occasionally someone would try to break the silence with the results of a ball game or a recent movie. Polite answers were mumbled in monosyllables. There was no blaming, and we kept a positive tone.

A box arrived with enough implants for six knees: left and right small, medium, and large femoral components.

The patient had a good outcome and neither the salesman nor I ever mentioned the mishap.

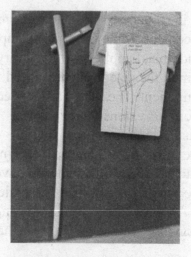

Internal Rod Fixation of a Femur

While I was performing a total knee replacement on a 69-year-old woman with advanced rheumatoid arthritis, the case was proceeding along as expected, although bones of patients with this type of arthritis are as soft and weak as balsa wood and break more easily than the average bone.

I had made a six-inch incision, turned over the patella, and flexed her knee to ninety degrees, effectively turning the knee inside out. I drilled a half-inch hole up into the center of the femoral canal and inserted an eight-inch rod. Then I slipped a stainless-steel cutting guide over the rod. Next, I inserted the oscillating saw blades through the slots on the guide and cut bone off the front and back of the femur. This prepared the bone for the trial femoral component designed to snug onto the bone like a large cap to provide the opportunity to test the fit before a permanent one is placed.

Carefully maintaining alignment, I tapped the trail cap onto the end of the freshly cut femur. I stopped to confirm alignment and proper contact on all cut surfaces from both the front and side views. Satisfied, I started to remove the trial component by tapping it gently.

The femur has two knobs (condyles) on the lower end, each about the size of a biscuit. Instead of staying put while I tapped, one broke off along with the trial component. Everyone in the room witnessed the potential catastrophe. All conversation stopped. I cursed under my breath, laid down my instruments, and folded my arms across my chest. What a predicament, I thought. What would Monaghan do?

I took a deep breath, removed the trial component, and rolled it around in my fingers. My options were few. Bone cement might have worked, but I decided to temporarily hold it in position with three small wires. I eyeballed the angle and drilled two holes one inch apart across the fracture, in preparation for a large compression screw. The threads engaged the bone on the far side of the fracture, allowing me to finish the total joint replacement with excellent long-term results.

~~~

During my early years, I was involved with two orthopedic studies with companies. I used each brand for fifty consecutive cases and was required to keep meticulous records, including five- and ten-year follow-ups. Reimbursement was only enough to cover the time involved for record-keeping. I learned quickly, especially about record-keeping. Limited time excluded my further involvement in total joint studies. Progress continues because of focused research by the orthopedic companies and surgeons dedicated to keeping detailed records.

CHAPTER 4

MISSION CLINIC

Gualaceo, Azuay Province, Ecuador – 1975

The urge to go on a mission trip lingered in the back of my mind for years. Although the idea of going to a distant land to work with the needy fueled my good intentions, the realities of work and time forced me to shelve my dreams. A physician presenting his medical mission trip to Ecuador during a national convention in 1994 captured Mary and my attention. Following a brief huddle at lunch, we committed to a two-week trip the following year. Although Mary lacked medical training, she had taught school and understood basic Spanish from her own high school studies. My responsibilities as an orthopedic surgeon were no better defined.

Local microbes had names like yellow fever, malaria, hepatitis, leprosy, and a plethora of toxigenic diarrhea-producing surprises. Ecuador had no health requirements, so I conferred with our Tulsa Health Department. Mary and I settled on shots for yellow fever and hepatitis to boost the immune system for about a month.

We were instructed to bring all the medications we could get out hands on, particularly antibiotics and anti-inflammatories. Because samples burdened the shelves of primary care physicians, they welcomed my visits. Most medications came in blister packs. To save space and weight, Mary and I spent evenings punching out thousands of pills to condense into smaller, well-labeled containers.

Volunteers were also asked to bring large duffel bags of donated surgery supplies, including reusable cloth drapes, disposable masks, caps, and shoes. Reusable gloves were not available in the United States, so we brought only disposable latex gloves. My concerns about customs proved unfounded, as we never saw an official, much less had our bags inspected.

~~~

Nine months later in April we flew into Quito, Ecuador. As the capital of Ecuador, at an elevation of 9,350 feet, it is the highest capital of the world, as well as the closest to the equator. Our arrival during the rainy season would mean daily rains in a climate of cool mornings and warm afternoons. The Andes Mountains dominated the western boundary and rainforests the eastern.

Waiting for our ride out of Quito, I favored the warmth of the sun, yet when I crossed the street into the shade of a building, the temperature dropped twenty degrees. A rusty school bus missing one side window picked us up and drove twenty miles to a town where our lodging had been arranged in a small hotel.

Along with Mary and I, the other sixteen members of our new team tried to be polite and visit, but the vertical snow-capped mountains claimed our attention. Mary took a remaining single seat on the aisle, and I took the one in front of her. Sitting in an aisle seat meant I had to lean over my seatmate to see the peaks.

Within minutes of leaving town and starting the Andes Mountain climb, the bus groaned along in second gear for the rest of the trip. Despite some drops over a mile to the bottom, I never saw a guardrail. As we switched to coming down the mountains, the greenery we'd viewed from the airport turned out to be gardens of corn. Arable land was so limited they planted corn up to doors of their homes. Everything was green up to the snow line. Clustered near fruit tree groves, houses built of cement and stucco were at various states of repair or construction. Most were small, about the size of a two-car garage back home. The water source came from the higher melting snow or small glaciers, and each year the appearance of an unexpected stream might bless a garden or wash it away.

The day was overcast with its promised afternoon rain. Because of the steep incline of the mountain, gravity dragged large amounts of mud down to our bus. Along the road we saw a lone woman walking uphill with a bundle of sticks piled high atop her head and more strapped on her back. A band around her head helped to balance the load, freeing her hands to carry more. Even from my seat on the bus, I could tell the bundles were too large for me to reach around. Surely, she had not mounted the load on her own back, but required assistance. I learned later the sticks were for cooking.

Mary leaned forward in her seat and tapped my shoulder. "If there is reincarnation," she murmured in my ear, "I don't want to come back as an Ecuadorian woman."

Walking uphill with a bundle on her back, another lady nursed a baby in one arm and carried a sack in the other.

I gathered our luggage, stepped off the bus, walked up a flight of stairs, and experienced immediate fatigue in the oxygen deprived air. Although we were on the equator, the high-altitude night temperature fell to forty-five degrees. The extra expense of heating our rooms at night was not included in the mission budget. I dressed as though I was going to sleep outdoors, with socks and a hoodie, and still I snuggled with Mary.

Back home in Tulsa, at an altitude of 722 feet, the stars twinkled, but in the cold of Ecuador's high elevations, they seemed to twinkle less. At lower altitudes, as the starlight passes through the atmosphere, the winds disturb the beam causing the stars to appear to twinkle. The Andes towered above most winds.

~~~

Our days at the mission clinic began with a knock on the door at five-thirty in the morning. Three of our group failed to make breakfast and orientation due to altitude sickness, which would abate in a day or two. The organizers scheduled me to screen patients in the clinic on Monday and Wednesday and perform surgery the remaining days, including Saturday. No one worked on Sunday.

Our program director stood sipping her coffee. "Never talk politics or religion," she said. "Those who came before you built a reputation and their work could be destroyed by a single innocent statement. Keep your religion and politics to yourself. This is not a program for recruitment. Complainers cannot be tolerated. Be open to eating strange foods. Eating strange foods should be a part of your experience. Because you will have unusual experiences here, you will never go all the way home."

Her comments evolved into a demand.

"On your last day, please leave behind everything possible, especially your dirty clothes." She settled her cup onto the table. "Shoes are needed, but nothing larger than size nine in men's shoes. Men here have small feet. You will receive specific orientations at your destinations. Your interpreters are good and know the locals. If in doubt about *anything*, ask them."

The local staff prepared sack lunches. By lottery four of our group won metal lunch boxes. I won a box with Batman and Robin on the side like the one I'd carried in the third grade. I wanted to believe it had once carried medicine or supplies from the U.S.

When Mary and I walked out to our respective minivans, I thought we were in a heavy fog. "This is a morning cloud we're in," our driver said. "If we drive slow, we'll be okay. The van going to the hospital will be in the clear in a few minutes, but the one up to the school will be in the cloud longer. We both know the way, even in a cloud."

Assigned to the eye-exam team of three, Mary was shuttled higher in the Andes to a single-room school. She learned the children were dismissed for the day because the school was reserved to fit reading glasses. An optometrist organized the exams for the eye team. Instead of using an eye chart with scrambled alphabet letters, Mary's team received instructions to splay three fingers as in an *E*.

The patient held a paper cup over one eye while he watched Mary with the other. With three fingers spread, Mary pointed up, straight across, and then down. The patient then pointed the same directions: up, across, or down.

Six shoeboxes of donated reading glasses sat in a line on a table and a patient sat behind each box. "They tried on every pair of glasses in the box," Mary said, "until they found one they liked. If not, they moved to the next box. When a patient found a fit, nothing needed to be said. They broke into a grin, looked at their palms then the back of their hands, especially their fingernails. They'd been out of focus for years."

The organizers shipped my crew in a different direction, to an old hospital built decades earlier by Communists and later deserted because of lack of staff. It rested at 9,820 feet in the small town of Gualaceo. When the Communists abandoned the country, Catholic nuns cared for the closed hospital and reopened it when visiting doctors and health caregivers came to town. Some days I rode with supplies in the back of a pickup and other days in a minivan. An interpreter, who was familiar with the locals, accompanied us.

At the hospital the teams lugged their gear inside and scoped out the facilities before going to their working destinations. The engineers took stock of the project list and set priorities for repairs. Our electrician won the longest list.

Despite being closed for years and opened now only a few weeks each year, the hospital still smelled like a hospital: a stale mixture of alcohol, medication and sickness, yet Lysol differentiated the surgery room.

Orientation specific to the hospital included operating solely on patients who required only minimal follow-up care, such as suture removal. No staged surgeries that would require additional surgery, such as screw or plate removal were scheduled. Because medical mission groups had been coming for years, the locals trusted the hospital and made long journeys to get there. We understood that building trust with the locals had required years to establish, and it was our responsibility to continue building on those relationships.

Additional briefing included a history of missions in that hospital which began eight years earlier and met strong opposition from the local dominating Catholic Church. The priests had interpreted the work of visiting health professionals as a covert operation to woo away church members, and they coached the Catholic community to avoid the caregivers. But church members in need of care visited the hospital through the back door. As the years passed, the priests realized the hospital and staff posed no threat and they began bringing church members to the hospital, praying with them, and giving last rites.

Our crew was the first one invited to tour their church, where they provided a sit-down dinner and a parade with music. The local surgery crew at the hospital spoke broken English, but we worked together understanding the common goal. While dinner cooked, we enjoyed a parade where the locals kept time with homemade instruments, including three drums and two flute-like instruments created from bamboo. Kids ran and skipped in front of and behind the band. With apparent pride, they showed us private rooms in the 140-year-old church that most of their members had never seen.

~~~

At the clinic I observed interactions between the locals. Once when two ladies visited with each other, the main talker stroked the other lady's hair. On a different occasion a mother placed her arm around the local interpreter's waist even though they were strangers. Outside the entrance two boys about eight years old held hands as they walked down the street.

Because we lacked the words to communicate, we were encouraged to touch the patients as much as practical. If the patient had a painful left elbow, I began by lightly cupping his right elbow, then slowly bending and extending it, setting the stage for him to give me access to his painful elbow.

I knew a caring touch spoke volumes to someone in pain. I asked *dolor*? as my fingers neared an area of pain. I added *mucho dolor o poco dolor?* Pressing on his normal arm, I repeated my questions as I touched and moved up his arm to eventually examine his elbow. When I'd established that I was going to be careful, I began working up his left arm to the painful elbow. Sometimes the patient answered with a nod or a headshake and occasionally by flinching, but never by pulling away.

Back home my patients' faith in the medical profession impressed me, which admittedly was reinforced by advertisements of new medications that always ended with "Ask your doctor." However, the patients in our clinic in Ecuador appeared to carry faith to a higher level, leading me to wonder if I might perform a surgery without anesthesia. What were the dynamics? Were they stoic, scared, appreciative? Even small children cooperated and seemed to lack fear. I held no false assumption that my presence had inspired the attitudes presented during our mission, and the permanent personnel confirmed that the profiles of the current patients matched those of previous mission trips.

After examining many men, I became aware of little to no hair on their arms. Although not important for patient care, I wondered if it had resulted from diet or altitude. Whether husband, wife or child, they all had round faces and black hair. Only children had short hair and all the women wore their hair down to their shoulders. Few had gray hair, probably from short life spans. Darker than olive, their skin was more like coffee with cream. A tall woman might reach five feet. Averaging about two inches taller, men weighed around 140 pounds. I never observed anyone obese, and I never saw anyone wearing glasses. By the time they reached thirty years of age, they had missing teeth, usually only two incisors, almost like a rite of passage. I understood from one of the local interpreters when a mother's milk dried up, they bottle-fed their baby with Coca-Cola because it was cheaper than milk.

Regardless of the terrain, the women wore shoes with about two-inch heels, even when carrying large bundles of sticks uphill or over uneven ground. An interpreter explained that for as long as he could remember, women had worn shoes with elevated heels. It was their culture.

Even without telephones or television, the public knew weeks ahead of time about our coming. I asked one of the English-speaking locals how the word spread. "We don't know how they find out," she said. "They know for miles around, even high in the Andes. We assume it's by word of mouth."

With an interpreter we screened patients and scheduled surgery for those we could help. When lunchtime arrived on our first day in the clinic, the interpreter closed the door on the patients waiting in line along the hall women had eight or more children, as menopause was the only effective basic birth control. No healthy, whole, or white teeth appeared to exist in all of Ecuador. Dentures accounted for the only normal appearing enamels, and even those were a coffee color. Hands were gnarled from weaving thousands of hats, and feet callused from a lifetime of contact with the earth, sans shoes.

The leader of the hospital team motioned toward another door. "Take your sack lunch and join the staff on the ground, next to the shaded wall outside," she said.

"What about those patients we left standing in line?" I asked.

"Don't worry about them," she said with a sympathetic tone. "They expect to wait. They have their straw hats to weave to sell for pennies per hat. Every girl learns how to weave a hat by the time she starts to school." She looked up and down the line. "Don't be tempted to buy a hat, because if you buy one hat, the others will expect you to buy one from them, too. They've been in line since yesterday and their families brought food." She paused and added, "Save your lunch sacks."

~~~

After lunch a ten-year-old boy presented with a bony mass on his right forehead. Big as a quarter, the bony mass protruded on the boy's forehead and had been present since early childhood. In addition to being teased, he could not wear a much-needed hat for shade at the high altitude. Even with beautiful brown skin, the boy's nose and cheeks revealed chronic sunburn from living at high elevation without wearing a hat. At a high altitude there was less atmosphere to filter the sun. I witnessed several children with chronic sunburn, especially on their noses. I scheduled surgery for the next day to remove the mass from his forehead.

His mother led him by the hand to the surgery room and left him at the door. She did not hesitate, smile, or show emotion. The surgery nurse, who did not speak Spanish, motioned him to come forward and patted the table for him to step up. Before he stepped up, the nurse gave him a big hug.

In the States we gave medication to relieve anxiety before going to surgery, but that luxury was not available to the poor people of Ecuador city, a hug from a caregiver did not replace medication, but I squatted and gave him a hug anyway. The rush was so fulfilling I became caught up in the moment and was tempted to give his mother a reassuring hug, but decided I might be violating her culture. The corners of her mouth flickered up breaking her somber face. We communicated without talking. Knowing neither our names nor speaking our language, the mother displayed the ultimate trust as she turned and walked away, leaving her son in our care. She joined her husband standing down the hall. We were later told, he could not tolerate coming closer to the surgery room. Looking at the crew's faces, I understood they felt the power of the hug. Everyone in the room had received a dose of trust and responsibility. Instructions, the boy stepped up to the stool, scooted back on the operating table and laid down expressionless. Without blinking his big beautiful brown eyes, he stared at the overhead lights. Full of trust. After watching his little heart beat through a thin, faded T-shirt, I felt compelled to kiss him on his check, an action unheard of back home. He never flinched. One of the nurses nodded. I represented everyone.

While the nurses and anesthesiologist prepared their equipment, I stood at his side, stroking his shoulder. After one quick glance at me, he blinked. I quite possibly was the first Caucasian he'd ever seen.

The anesthesiologist held a mask above the boy's face and spoke with a soft voice in a tongue foreign to the boy. He stroked the boy's hair and shoulder with his left hand, while slowly lowering the mask over his mouth and nose.

The possibility of skin cancer threatened the child on the table before me, simply because he couldn't wear a hat. I held the skills to perform a simple, yet critical, surgery. But I'd never operated on a skull. After he was sound asleep, I made an inch-and-a-half transverse incision across his head, exposing the hard mass. I then proceeded to uncover the thin layer of life-giving tissue covering the bone. I cut through the protective layer, about as thick as an apple skin, and peeled it back, exposing the bone.

I used an ordinary hammer and chisel. For a similar surgery back home, I would have used an expensive mallet and curved chisels of six to eight sizes, then finish with a power burr to smooth and contour the bone. But that day I had only one chisel, about a half-inch wide. With the edge of the chisel at the base of the mass, I began tapping lightly to test the hardness of the bone.

The boy's hard bone represented healthy bone, further confirming the mass was likely benign. As my chisels passed through the bone, the deeper layers peeled off in ribbons with the consistency of pine-wood. When I shaved the bone down to the contour of his forehead, I smoothed the final surface with an ordinary carpenter's file, the same file I used to sharpen the chisel before surgery. I trimmed the excess skin with scissors and closed the wound with stitches. In one week, a nurse would remove the stitches.

As I finished my first surgery, I said the traditional thank you to the operating room staff, then turned, pulled off my disposable latex gloves and dropped them in a small trash can inside the surgery room.

Without a word, a local nurse picked the used gloves out of the trash. Back home, saving bloodstained gloves ranked with washing and reusing paper towels, Kleenex, and toilet paper. Embarrassed, I never made the same mistake again. Instead, after peeling off disposable gloves, I laid them on the table. With surgery concluded for the day, I lingered and found an excuse to enter their cleaning room. I stepped quietly inside the door and remained unnoticed as the nurse scrubbed and washed the blood from the sheets and gowns, which would be steri-lized later. As she washed the gloves, she turned them inside out several times. Finally, she filled each glove with air from her mouth, twisted its top, and dunked it under water looking for bubbles indicating a hole. Those disposable gloves would be used again and again until bubbles appeared. I backed quietly out of the room.

~~

If a patient and family arrived a day early, they staked their claim in the line and followed an unwritten etiquette of maintaining that position, even if required to remain overnight. While they stood, sat, squatted, and visited for hours, the line adapted to waiting and developed a community of caring. If a woman waited with a baby, she held priority over others, including those in pain. I would not have been surprised to see a stranger nurse the baby. A lone person was offered food from families in line. Time was not relevant to the group, and I never saw a watch. "They do not have a concept of hours in a day," our interpreter explained, "and therefore they do not understand eight o'clock in the morning. They only know it means sometime before midday."

On the tenth day I ate a late lunch with Maria, the interpreter. As we sat leaning against the shaded wall, I began unwrapping my Spam sandwich, but then stalled with a thought.

"This has been one heck of an experience for me. How do the locals see us?"

"They are so appreciative of what you do for them, but the surgery is not the only issue. There's more. Much more. And you cannot recognize it."

I shifted a chunk of food inside my cheek. "What is?"

"Hope." She spoke without hesitation. "You folks show what an education brings. The younger ones understand more than their parents."

"And there is more?"

"Caring." Maria went on to explain that those who come provide a service and do a good job, were viewed as interesting and unusual. "A few see it as an adventure and go home with bragging rights about their work." She nodded as though to reassure herself. "They've earned it." The nod drifted into a headshake. "But they never come back. The locals really want to know that you care enough to come back. That's the difference. Few care enough to come back."

"I'll be back."

In medical school I had studied and viewed pictures of classic yet rare diseases, but seldom did I come across one in practice. However, in the clinic in Ecuador I saw more children with six toes or six fingers than in all the years of my practice.

A child with six fingers could not wear a glove. A child with six toes must cut out the side of any shoe, which resulted in their being treated as an outcast. If a child had a problem with both feet or both hands, I had to decide where to operate first. I had one chance to do the most good.

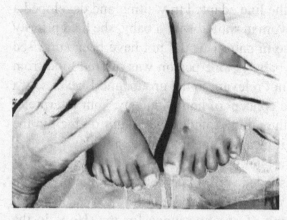

Six Toes on Each Foot

Removing a sixth finger involved more than the digit. The supporting long bone, the metacarpal, in the hand also needed to be removed. The same principle applied to the foot where I removed the extra toe and the supporting long bone, the metatarsal.

~~~

One morning a wife and two daughters brought a man into the clinic on a homemade stretcher of bamboo and woven leaves, lightweight but remarkably strong. X-rays revealed a fracture of his right femur at a distorted angle of twenty degrees and the fracture edges overlapped one-and-a half inches. The interpreter understood the injury occurred about a month before. Because patients did not use calendars except for keeping track of Sundays, the time since his injury was vague. Without correction, the man's fracture would result in a deformity that would forever keep him walking with a marked limp and eventually destroy his hip and knee joints from the abnormal stress angles.

I explained to the interpreter how I was going to try to straighten the man's leg with a metal plate and screws that could break or get infected. I added he might have a limp. The interpreter turned to the patient and his family and said something in Spanish that sounded like four words.

"That was fast. What did you say to the patient?"

"You're having surgery tomorrow."

When I reviewed the inventory of bone plates, I discovered only a twelve-inch, twelve-hole plate, and a two-inch plate. The deformity called for an eight-inch, eight-hole plate. Using an ordinary hacksaw from a carpenter's toolbox, I cut down the longer one to eight inches. Then I filed off the sharp corners with the same file I'd used for smoothing the boy's head. The progressive twinge of doubt entered my mind. I had no one to call and no instruction book to read.

I took a deep breath and made the incision on the side of his thigh and dissected down through the muscles until I came to the bone. Using the same chisel that I'd used on the boy's head, I pounded and cracked the healing crooked bones.

His muscles were contracted because the bone overlapped the muscles and tendons in his thigh. The procedure was imperative because if the leg was overlapping, his leg could not be stretched back to its normal length. I began having reservations about fixing the one-month-old fracture. Being off it as much as a week would be critical, and one week might be lost in translation. If I could not stretch his leg to the normal end-to-end length, I would need to saw off small slices of bone from both ends until I could pull the ends together. In anticipation, I requested the carpenter hacksaw sterilized.

Attempting to lengthen his leg was fraught with possible complications, including permanent nerve injury, which would further cripple him and render his leg useless. I needed feedback from the surgery crew, but they looked at me as though I had all the answers. I studied the x-rays on the wall, and swallowed hard.

Once again, I yearned for my equipment from back home. In Tulsa I would have placed the patient on a mechanical fracture table that could pull the overlapping fracture to length and alignment. However, like all others on our medical mission, I worked with the tools at hand.

We turned the patient onto his side and maintained his position with multiple rolls of tape. I did some powerful pulling. We washed, scrubbed, and draped his thigh.

What the hell am I doing here, I wondered. For the second time today, I'm doing a surgery I've never heard of.

As I expected, he began bleeding. Fortunately, the surgery room provided cautery whereby I could burn the ends of small bleeders and tie the bigger ones. Both bone ends were easy to locate because they were almost next to the skin. With his knee bent next to my abdomen, I wrapped my right arm around his leg and began pulling.

As a kid playing with tent poles, I figured out the mechanical advantage of pushing down if the pole legs were far apart. That day in surgery, I repeated my childhood play. I held the ends of the fractured 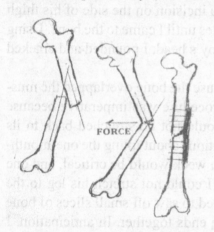 bone like two tent poles and slowly pushed down, applying progressive pressure. The peak of the angle rested in my right palm with my left hand stacked on top. The bone ends came together at about twenty degrees, and the mechanical advantage favored me. I silently coached myself to be patient and allow time for the muscles and tendons to fatigue and stretch. I budgeted fifteen minutes of pushing.

Fractured Femur with Plate and Screws

This is crud.

Pressing down, I looked around the room for encouraging eyes. No one even blinked. They look like they think I know what I'm doing.

When I fatigued, the assistant took a turn applying his body weight on the apex of the joining bones. Which would fatigue first? The surgery crew or the patient's muscles and tendons? We continued pressing down. Minutes dragged. No one talked. As the patient's muscles and tendons fatigued, the apex lowered. The muscles and tendons stretched until they were taut as fiddle strings. I thought they might vibrate from tension. Fifteen minutes inched past. The contracted muscles and tendons finally released.

I needed a slight bow in the plate to match the normal contour of the femur. After laying the plate next to the femur, I turned to the instrument table and took sterilized pliers and a pipe wrench to bend the plate in increments. After using a hand drill to create eight screw holes in the bone, I secured the plate to the femur with four screws on each side of the fracture.

I bandaged his thigh, anxious to check his pulse on the top of his foot. If the pulse was good in his foot, then the main blood vessel in his thigh was open and working well. Until he was well awake, I couldn't confirm nerve sensation by scratching his foot. At the time I applied the plate, his main nerve and blood vessels were behind the field where I had worked. Therefore, I would not know until later if I'd pulled the artery apart or overstretched the nerve.

I closed the incision, applied a dressing, and transferred him to a gurney.

Standing beside him, I placed my right index, middle and ring fingers over the artery on top of his foot. I waited to feel a pulse. Nothing. The silence around the gurney was louder than a drum roll.

"Hand me some pillows to place under his leg."

I prepared to take any action that might help, including draining the slightest hint of swelling from his leg.

"What do you want to do about the next case?" The anesthesiologist understood my dilemma.

"Let's go ahead and start the next case," I said, knowing everyone wanted to finish the day.

Although anxious about my patient in recovery, I drained an old abscess on another man's foot, trimmed away the dead muscle and skin, and left open the hole. Weighing the patient's options, I gambled that the hole would heal from the inside out. Throughout the abscess case, I fretted to check the previous patient's foot for a pulse. If the pulse did not return, my options were to leave it alone and hope for the best or return him to surgery to attempt an impossible repair. I would have to take out the plate and start cutting off both broken ends until I could bring the bones end-to-end and apply the plate on a shortened femur. Perhaps neither idea would work.

If blood did not return as indicated by a pulse, his leg would die. He would then be better off if he'd never come to the hospital but stayed in the mountains and crawled under his house. If his leg died, removing his dead leg was more than simply cutting it off. Amputation included a step-by-step removal, but more important, a step-by-step closing of the flaps. But when the leg began to smell in a week or two, there'd be no medical personnel available. Back home I did not face so many variables, and the usual decision-making algorithm did not fit his case.

When I finished the abscess surgery, I removed my gown and gloves in a hurry and headed down the hall to determine the fate of the man's leg. Lining up my three fingers, I searched the top of his foot for a pulse and waited. Nothing. I generated enough nervous energy that I could have powered the hospital.

"You check for a pulse." I spoke with a guarded voice, stepping aside to make room for the nurse. She placed three fingers on the top of the patient's foot and waited. "I feel something."

"Are you sure?" I said in hurry, as though the pulse might go away, and nudged my way beside the patient. "Let me feel. I feel something," I adjusted my fingers on his foot. Silence saturated the room. "Here, you feel it again." I deferred to the nurse, seeking confirmation.

I'd heard that a female could feel a pulse before a male because of their softer fingers. I wanted to believe it.

"Yes, it's here. Right under my fingers." Without looking up, she continued pressing her fingers on his foot.

To confirm the good news, I again took a turn. I savored the pulse on his foot that beat a regular rhythm of life-giving blood to his leg. However to test whether the nerve reacted to simple pinprick, I was forced to wait overnight because of the anesthesia.

The following morning before I was fully awake, the patient with the recovered pulse dominated my thoughts. I was the first one off the van and went directly to his room with an interpreter. For a baseline, I scratched his good foot with a pin.

"Does this feel sharp?" asked the interpreter in Spanish.

He nodded. I moved to his right leg. My heart quickened as I dragged the pin along the top of his foot.

"Does this feel sharp?" asked the interpreter.

"Sí."

"Tell him to move his foot up and down." I sucked in a deep breath.

The foot moved up and down. I let out my breath. The relief was so great I eased into a bedside chair hoping to camouflage my relief.

They knew.

I accepted my first cup of coffee of the day.

During his leg surgery, his family wove and tied together crutches of a remarkable tan and green pattern, all from bamboo, in one afternoon. Under normal conditions, the patient would remain non-weight bearing on his right leg for two to four months and serial x-rays would be used to confirm healing before any weight bearing was allowed. We had to trust that the patient and his family understood he could not bear weight for three months.

The mother and daughters also wove hats while waiting. Because I was as pale as a glass of milk and burned easily, I bought a hat from the wife. My head was bigger than their general market, and even though it sat high on my head, I was glad for the hat. The family snickered.

He left the hospital the second day after surgery with only aspirin for his pain.

Fatigued from the intensity of the day, our crew filed in to the minivan. I chose a seat next to a window, the softest seat in town. A seat so comfortable that whenever the driver hit or dodged potholes in the gravel road, I did not feel jostled as I had coming to the hospital. Normally the snow-capped peaks on the right side and the extreme deep valleys on the left captured my attention. Instead, I relived the day with the happy families who had waited for hours, maybe days. I failed to see the mountains, but focused on the frugal living conditions where the locals struggled to grow enough food on such steep hillsides. I didn't see any cattle, only goats, leaving me to wonder if cows could live on such steep slopes.

Once again, we passed lone women walking uphill with large bundles of sticks on their backs.

I usually joined the chatter on the crooked thirty-minute mountain-hugging ride in the scenic Andes. But not that day. The day's work had exposed me to the weight of trust and the charge of building relationships. No one questioned my decisions about which stranger I could help and which I could not. Decision-making was my sole responsibility.

I pondered how the nuns accomplished so much with so little.

My spirit grew heavy as I recalled instructing the interpreter to tell a mother, father or child that I could not help a painful joint. The interpreter never needed to explain or repeat the bad news. Without expression, patients accepted their fate and walked away.

Deep in my own reflections, I became aware of the absence of chatter. Even the talkers were not talking. Everyone appeared sedated or under a spell. The silence did not represent fatigue, because no one was sleeping. A quick survey around the bus revealed unfocused stares, as though everyone had entered an inner world unaware of the world around them.

What about Mary's day? If her rewards were half as intense as mine, I wanted to hear about each one with no details left out.

We'd been the givers of care for the day, but what was given us? Nothing in our pockets. No trinkets, no souvenirs. Instead, we carried home the satisfaction of making a lasting difference in the lives of strangers, and the lessons learned would last a life.

Our orientation leader was right. I would not be going all the way home. But did I care enough to return? Had I made an irrational commitment? Should I have talked with Mary first? Should I even mention my knee jerk commitment?

During our efforts at the mission, I never saw a patient or family member cry. However, when alone, I wanted to squeeze out a tear for all those I could not help, and I yearned for confirmation from a peer that I'd made the right decisions. My shoulders slumped with fatigue.

Staring out the window, I sang along in silence with Louis Armstrong, remembering the comforting last words of an old favorite:

I hear babies crying, I watch them grow
They'll learn much more than I'll ever know
And I think to myself,
What a wonderful world.

CHAPTER 5

ORTHOPEDIC PRACTICE

Tulsa, Oklahoma

1976-1987

My rotation of call schedules separated me from my partners. We were never in the same surgery suite to share the challenge of a new procedure. I wanted someone on my level to share the joys in the challenges of daily surgical practice, and I yearned for lively and engaged discussions reviewing the results of surgery. I missed the camaraderie and academic discussions at conferences. As a resident, my interactive conversations with other doctors and surgeons had generated a better work environment. I screwed up my courage and proposed a new idea at an office meeting.

"I would like to look into applying for an orthopedic residency training program," I said at our monthly meeting. "I think we have the volume and variety."

"I don't think you understand how much paperwork that will entail," Campion said. "That requires time and energy devoted to the residents. And don't forget, we would be training our own competition."

"The resident would be the one on call, which would be a bonus for us," I explained.

When they didn't squelch the idea, I walked away with a spring in my step, anticipating having young and enthusiastic orthopedic residents in our daily work arena.

From the beginning I vowed that the new training program would be different from the one I'd experienced. I envisioned a program that instructed from a position of support and encouragement instead of criticism. The new program would expect a resident to support opinions based on accepted literature and to discuss the points with rational arguments. Emphasis would be on supporting the orthopedic residents, who would be working long hours.

~~~

The program application process required two years and an on-sight inspection. The program did not pay the teaching surgeons a salary or reimbursement for expenses, but it provided the satisfaction of being around enthused doctors. Besides, I harbored a need to pay back to the profession what it had given me.

I coached myself to be mindful that these students were not twenty-two-year-old college graduates but adults, mostly in their late twenties and early thirties; some would be almost as old as I was. I reviewed and cleared the proposed program with the other orthopedic surgeons on staff. The residents would become my extended family. Perhaps I could become their Monaghan.

When the training program was approved, I drove home with a feel-good grin.

"Mary, get ready for company. We're going to grow a new family."

I didn't have a Romano's restaurant, but even better, I had access to a good selection of meeting rooms. The residents gradually decorated the orthopedic meeting room I'd selected with anatomy posters, and I now had a new cabinet to display my collection of orthopedic tools and implants that I'd collected over the years.

~~~

Until medical school, I had assumed a blood test was the magic bullet, revealing all I needed to know about a patient to diagnose the health problem. Looking at blood under a microscope translated to high-level science and accuracy, or so I thought. X-rays were equally important in making an early diagnosis. My professors had known differently, however, emphasizing the value of an accurate patient history to determine a diagnosis. Experience had taught me that their method was accurate more than eighty percent of the time, and now it was my duty to pass on this critical knowledge to new residents.

To emphasize the importance of taking an accurate patient history as a crucial initial step in the diagnosis process, I explained to the new residents that if I took into consideration the patient's age, duration of complaint, pattern of pain, and precipitating event, I could usually come up with a probable diagnosis before drawing blood or looking at an x-ray.

To emphasize the point, if I had a student or resident with me in my office, we read the history from the chart hanging on the door and guessed the diagnosis before entering the room. For example if a forty-two-year-old patient said his hand was going to sleep, especially his thumb, index and middle fingers, and he had to shake his hand for relief, the diagnosis was carpel tunnel syndrome. X-rays only added value to rule out surprises, such as a foreign object in a hand.

For over twenty-seven years, along with orthopedic staff, I met with residents to review x-rays of the week, and sometimes host a guest lecture. The rewards of watching the residents in training trumped the paperwork required. They never complained or whined, but worked hard, learned their craft, and made me proud. *Run me harder, coach,* should have been their motto.

As our program developed and news of our residency spread we fine-tuned our application process and the quality of the residents improved. I wanted to be a friend to these young professionals but not a buddy. I understood that if I respected them, I would earn their respect. Long ago I had told myself I would never embarrass them.

Throughout my years of involvement in our resident program, only one resident disappointed me. His technical skills were good, but his interaction with the personnel did not improve. He passed the selection process, but he always gave an excuse as to why he was late or in conflict with the nursing staff. Our department members met with him one-on-one over the four years. His conduct was never enough to dismiss him. I bragged and rooted for him in public, especially after he performed surgery. We were never prepared to dismiss a resident. Like the parent of a wayward child, I continued to fret what action I should take with the young wayward resident. I began taking hypertension medication. Within two years of practice, he was divorced and asked to leave a hospital staff. I kept up with him through coffee talk as he moved through practice, locations, and wives.

~~~

When I took on the responsibilities of being a designated trainer, I knew the position came without compensation, but I viewed it as an opportunity to pay back Monaghan and the other orthopedic surgeons who had allowed me to operate on their patients and learn from them.

The designated trainer must have not only a passion for teaching, coaching, and interaction, but must biannually attend a weekend course focused on training techniques for orthopedic residents. Every year the course was taught in Chicago and coordinated by an experienced lecturer with a PhD in orthopedic training.

The method taught by the PhD emphasized that being an active role model was more effective than lecturing or providing verbal instruction. He reminded us we were not dealing with college students but highly motivated adults wanting to learn and nurture their careers while balancing family needs. These new residents were enthusiastic, and despite having the responsibility of spouses and young children, they were willing to dedicate years of their lives to developing a specialty in orthopedics.

Although I, too, had made these sacrifices, I still found it astounding that someone would willingly make this kind of commitment.

In Chicago, the training instructor explored how to motivate orthopedic residents, recognize depression, deal with personal conflicts, and know when to seek professional consultation. For the first time in their careers, they were not graded or ranked but only issued progress reports.

Six active orthopedic surgeons worked on the orthopedic selection committee, and I served as one of them. For two open positions in the program, the number of applicants each year ranged from 50 - 60. The first screening would eliminate about ten percent because their forms were incomplete or not legible. Average grades were not an absolute reason for rejection if the remaining parts of an application were impressive. Our committee understood grades were important, but the applicant must first be a team player.

As the committee reviewed the applicants, we discovered the most effective network resource was the residents in our program. On several occasions, we had not selected the semifinalists for interviews because we needed more than the information in the packet.

"May we look at the list?" said the chief resident. He pointed to a photo. "He was two years behind me. I can call a good friend who is in his class and he will tell me straight about him. I can get more information over the phone than you can get off his application."

Our committee postponed the decision for a week, providing the current residents time to make calls and gather more information concerning the applicants. By networking, the residents eliminated another third of the applicants from our list, and only three on the remaining list received outstanding recommendations by their peers. The residents had bonded to protect their program. Two weeks later, the committee interviewed twelve applicants.

Driving home after the interviews, I reflected on the informal phone call I had received from Monaghan that had changed my life forever. By current standards my acceptance into the training program was simple and crude. On reflection, I was embarrassed to have felt special.

The final selection day drained my energy and I didn't sleep well that night, aware that our decisions had dramatically changed lives of the few applicants we had accepted in to the program, as well as those who were not accepted.

I felt like a phony with a double standard. I was lucky to have been born when selection was almost by default. These applicants were not lucky, but each had earned the right to be considered. Monaghan, long deceased, would have understood. When I was their age I was unsure and riddled with anxiety, but these applicants presented themselves with confidence. Had they practiced or been coached for the interview? They all wore a coat and a tie. I didn't even own a suit when I'd applied; I was wearing a pair of black wingtips shoes I'd bought my sophomore year in college that had been resoled several times with several heel replacements as well. How did these applicants pay for travel halfway across the country for an interview?

As the orthopedic program chairman, it was my responsibility to oversee their program and the quality of training. After twenty-seven years, I turned the program over to a peer. Thereafter, I functioned as one of the staff's orthopedic surgeons.

Reflecting on my career in orthopedics, I wanted to be certain Monaghan would have been proud he'd chosen the second person on the list.

~~~

My career as an orthopedic surgeon required me to be a teacher *and* a student—sometimes both in the same day. Although I was licensed to practice a broad range of surgeries, I didn't always have the expertise and training specific to new surgical procedures that had recently been developed.

For instance, I had years of practice behind me, but I was still lacking experience with advanced hand surgery. Every time I went to a large city for a convention or orthopedic course, I copied the names and addresses of anyone in the yellow pages who promoted themselves as hand surgeons. I drafted letters regarding my interest in training in hand surgery, and to make myself an attractive candidate, I told them I would work for free. My two orthopedic partners also recognized the need for a hand surgeon in our practice and agreed to subsidize me for the duration of the training if I was accepted as a trainee.

Tulsa continued to have only one fellowship-trained hand surgeon; the entire U. S. only had five fellowship training programs, and at forty-one years of age I applied to all five. I wanted to think that my age and overall experience gave me an edge on the other applicants.

I was accepted into the program based in Michigan. When hand programs were first being developed, the training required only six months. However, as knowledge and procedures expanded, fellowship programs were increased to one year. I entered a six-month fellowship.

Even with my advanced training, there were still procedures that required more instruction. Carpal tunnel syndrome was an orthopedic problem that had been around since the building of the pyramids. A wrist splint that limited motion was the first step in treatment, but if pain continued a curved two-inch incision in the palm and over the nerve would usually release the pressure with a good outcome.

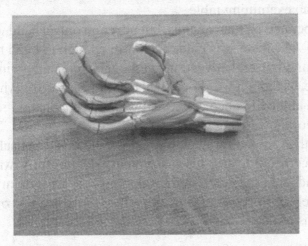

A Teaching Model Almost Identical to the Hand Amputation

Orthopedic manufacturers entered the market to promote their instrument for treating carpal tunnel syndrome. However, the steps of any instrument needed to be followed in detail. To promote the safety of a new product, a surgical company would not sell the new instruments unless the surgeon had gone through a surgical orientation offered by the company. I signed up for an orientation, understanding that the salesman would come to my office to train me.

As agreed, when I received a package sent by special delivery I was to notify the local sales representative. The box was large enough to hold a bowling ball but was full of Styrofoam packed with dry ice around a human hand.

I stared at the hand, resting palm up, and wondered about its history and how it had toiled. According to instructions, I was to discard all frozen material and place the hand back into the empty box to permit it to thaw overnight.

At the end of the following day the sales representative came to my office and instructed me how his instrument worked on the cadaver hand. All day I was uncomfortable knowing a hand waited for me. When the office closed and the personnel had gone, the salesman and I worked at an examining table.

I had operated on many hands, but never on only a hand, unattached to a human. The hand was cold, but warm enough to bend the fingers. The lone hand poised between us on the table created an inexplicable atmosphere, as though we should whisper or be aware of what we said. I wondered at the life once connected with this hand, and I saw signs it had once worn a wedding band.

In less than fifteen minutes we had finished, and the salesman declared me certified to use his instrument. He carefully wrapped the thawed hand and replaced it in the shipping box. Despite my curiosity I did not feel comfortable asking him what would become of the hand.

That was too personal.

~~~

At that time in Tulsa, if a patient entered the ER with an amputated finger or hand, no one on our staff or anyone in the city, was trained to reattach it. Orthopedic surgeons understood that without micro instruments, amputated extremities could not be reattached. First, our carpenter-like tools were too large to manipulate small arteries, veins, and nerves. Second, the anatomy was too small to visualize without magnification. The required sutures were no bigger than a hair and too small to tie into a simple square knot. Eye surgeons had worked with microscopes for years, but no other surgery field had recognized a need for them.

An artery carries oxygen-rich blood from the heart to the arms and legs and returns through the veins where it enters the lungs to pick up another load of oxygen. To save an amputated arm or leg, blood flow must be returned within hours. Microsurgery is required to make it happen. Vital organs such lungs, heart, and brain can be permanently damaged after a few minutes without proper oxygen-rich blood; a limb, however, can survive for four to six hours. Patient age, co-injuries, and iced transportation of the severed limb affect the viability of the limb. Qualifying amputations are those with smooth, well-defined edges, and for these select situations microsurgical techniques made the impossible, possible.

Progress began when curious orthopedic surgeons borrowed instruments from eye surgeons to explore the potential of reattachment. Practicing with the right equipment, surgeons improved their rate of success.

An orthopedic journal announced a micro-vascular course in Denver. The course was full at twenty-two students. I registered and paid the fee, which included a microscope, toy-like microscopic instruments, and a live white rat. Each microscope had two viewing eyepieces, allowing two surgeons to view the field simultaneously. The lighted operative field was no larger than a nickel.

The instructor began his lecture with the dismal history of attempts to reattach limbs. Because previously all reattachments failed, surgeons learned not to waste valuable time trying with an arm, hand, or finger. We listened to lectures for two days before moving to the lab.

The femoral artery and vein in the groin of an adult lab rat are the same diameter as in an adult male finger, no larger than a pencil lead. Proctors sedated each rat, injected local anesthetic, and then severed the rat's groin artery and vein. The rat needed to stay alive with its heart pumping to confirm repairs a success. Successful or not, the rats were sacrificed.

We were charged with repairing the artery and vein in ninety minutes. Learning to use a microscope and microscopic instruments was tedious, exhausting work. Assistants walked the room coaching but not assisting. Most of the students completed a reattachment with satisfactory blood flow in the allotted time. When the class concluded at the rat lab, we gathered at the bar to congratulate others and brag on ourselves.

~~~

Twelve years into my practice and two months after the micro vascular course, I was walking out of the surgery suite when I received a call from the ER.

A young man lay on a cart with a drape across his body covering his hands. I removed the drape. His severed left hand was cradled in a bloody pool in his right hand. The amputation crossed his wrist with only a half-inch strip of skin stretched between. An agitated co-worker spilled the story between sobs and pointed out the jerry-rigged tourniquet—the patient's belt.

The carpenter had been using a hand-held power saw to cut off a corner of a plywood sheet. He'd held the panel in place across his knee with his left hand ahead of the saw. Using his dominate right hand to push and guide the saw, he kept his index finger on the trigger. The spinning blade struck a nail in the wood, kicked back and up, leaping out of the wood. The saw traveled forward cutting off his left hand above his wrist. The sequence had happened before he could release the trigger, faster than the flip of a switch.

The surgery crew wheeled him to the operating room and placed him under general anesthesia within fifteen minutes of arrival at the hospital. With the patient lying on his back, I held his left arm in the air, draining as much blood back into his body as possible. The orthopedic resident assisting me, Dr. James Harrington, began wrapping his arm with a four-inch-wide elastic bandage from his wrist to his shoulder, squeezing the remaining blood out of his arm into his body.

Orthopedic surgeons working on an arm or leg had an advantage over other surgeons because a tourniquet can be applied above the area of surgery to keep the operative field dry of blood. After the wrap reached tourniquet level between elbow and shoulder, the anesthesiologist, Dr. William Sturdevent, turned the switch to inflate the tourniquet well above normal blood pressure. When the surgery ended and the tourniquet released, the arm quickly filled with blood, but ended with spurts at the amputation. I couldn't figure a way to save the lost blood. The ends needed to be preserved as much as possible. Permitting them to bleed was contrary to normal surgery.

No one in the room had any experience with reattaching a human limb, especially me. I was supposed to lead the effort but had only the rat-vessel-reattachment for experience. Working on the rat did not compare to the stress of being responsible for the future of this man's hand. In the lab I had practiced on one artery and vein that were stable. Now I faced both bones severed, along with cut nerves and more than fifteen tendons severed.

"Start the clock." I said knowing I had two hours in which to work, the longest his arm could tolerate without blood. Then I would need to release the tourniquet, allow the life-giving blood to flush his limb, and start the process over. I had no idea how long the procedure would take, but silent stress in the room communicated commitment to be there until the task concluded, whether results were good or bad.

Even the slightest movement could cause the micro sutures to tear through the artery or vein walls. Because of time constraints, I elected to stabilize the larger of two wrist bones, the radius. We pulled the bone ends together and applied a plate with two screws on each side of the gap.

The time from amputation to reattachment of an artery and vein was critical, but a nerve repair could be delayed until the end of a case or delayed for days. The limb must be reattached within four to five hours, maybe six. No one knew. The limb begins dying without blood.

Time, time, my enemy is time. Shit.

Harrington had no experience with a surgical microscope, only a simple microscope in medical school where students looked at non-living cells. I quickly taught him how to use a microscope and assist me while I was learning how to reattach a hand.

If the patient lost his hand, it would be because of the amputation by the saw. If he lost his arm up to the tourniquet above his elbow, it would be my fault because I misjudged how much tourniquet time his arm could endure.

95

Another surgeon may have recognized the impossible, clipped the small amount of skin between the amputated parts, rounded off the two wrist bones and closed the skin in one procedure. The patient would have left the hospital in three or four days with no one criticizing the surgeon. Waiting nervously, I began second-guessing myself during the ten minutes of tourniquet release. The world was full of second-guessers and Monday morning quarterbacks who would be glad to tell me what I should have done, including not to accept the case. But there was no-where to send my patient. When I determined the plate on the radius was secure, I began my first reattachment without benefit of practice or an experienced assistant. No one in the room had ever seen a reattachment.

"How much time have we used?" I asked Dr. Studevant, the anesthesiologist.

"One hour, forty-seven."

He did not need to remind me I had about fifteen more minutes to get a blood flow or—or what? Should I continue to work in the face of starving the hand of blood?

I needed only one more suture on the front wall of the vein, but I had delayed it to the last because it was the easiest to reach. I couldn't help thinking it was simple in the rat lab, but a damn difficult surgery for a beginner in real life.

The room needed a leader. "Once we hit two hours, call out the time used every five minutes."

"Five minutes," said Dr. Sturdevant.

If I could complete the final stitch in ten more minutes, it was worth the potential risk of depriving the muscles of oxygen. Under the scope I brought the tip of the needle slowly into the field from my right side. The side of my hand always rested on the table to eliminate any non-productive moves. The magnification was sensitive enough to pick up the movement of my hand caused by my heartbeat. Each artery and vein needed only four stitches: one at the three, six, nine, and twelve o'clock positions. However, after only two micro-sutures in place, the time limit was up.

I released the tourniquet to flood his arm for ten minutes. Blood did not flow past the amputation but pumped like water out of a cut garden hose. Ten minutes of watching him bleed seemed closer to ten hours. I could only wait. I mopped up blood and washed clots from the surgery area. I repeated wrapping and squeezing blood out of his arm up to the tourniquet, running the risk of tearing loose the microscopic sutures. Then I squeezed the blood from his arm back into his body.

"Inflate the tourniquet and start the clock," I said. One suture had pulled loose because of the manipulation.

At the second two-hour limit, I released the tourniquet and flushed his arm with fresh blood. Because I had not completed the artery and vein repairs, no blood passed to the hand.

On the third two-hour flush, I had only the minimum of four sutures in each artery and vein, plus a stabilizing plate and screws on the radius of the wrist.

I did not yet plate the second bone because my time needed to be focused on establishing blood flow. The first plate held the radius enough to work on the critical blood vessels.

Through the microscope I saw the arc of fatigue by the progressive tremor of my fingers. Willing the tremor to cease long enough to pass one more suture was no longer possible. Only Harrington could see the tremor and whispered, "You're doing fine. We're out of time and I bet your sutures will hold."

With great anxiety, I released the tourniquet. All in the room remained silent, eyes focusing on the flat artery as it filled. The welcomed normal pulse throbbed across the repair sight. Until I took a deep inhalation, I did not know I had been holding my breath.

Six hours and three tourniquet releases had passed. Harrington and I were fatigued from straining over the unfamiliar microscope. The stool had a low back I leaned against for the first time. Using gentle pressure, I packed the wound and did not close the skin, so as not to apply too much pressure on the swollen muscles. The lacerated muscles showed signs of early swelling from the original injury, aggravated by my surgical manipulation.

Time. I've got have more time.

More surgery remained, including plating the second bone, repairing nerves, muscles, and tendons in the face of continued swelling.

When could I return him to surgery? Tomorrow? Two to three days? The longer the skin was not pulled closed, the odds of infection increased. I elected to lightly pack the open wound with wet gauze. We elevated his hand to drain swelling and return him to surgery on Wednesday.

Stopping outside the waiting room door, I prepared to talk to his family. I rehearsed my options. *Was it a success? Would I say I had reattached his hand.? Would I have to bring him back to surgery if a finger turns dark from a clot? Was the tip of a finger turning dark while I talked to the family? Do I say I am tired? Will they wonder why I didn't call another doctor?*

Pulling back my slumped shoulders, I took a deep breath and explained to the family that blood was flowing into his fingers when I left the room, but small clots could stop the flow at any time. Every hour that passed with the tips of the fingers remaining pink was a bonus. If the fingers stayed pink for hours, then days, the outcome looked good. "I will know in three-four weeks if the bone is healing," I said to them, "but the nerves will require months to regenerate." The rest of my diagnosis was harder to deliver. The range of motion and function would improve over the next year, but he would not have the strength or sensory processing needed to be a carpenter.

I left the family, turned left into the recovery room, and lay down, staring at the ceiling. "If I fall asleep, wake me in fifteen minutes," I said to a nurse who pulled back a corner of the curtain.

The rest of the day I strained to see if the tips of any of my patient's fingers were turning dark, the first sign of blockage. If they were, what were my options? Did I try to loosen the dressing or take him back to surgery—and do what? I felt had no viable options. I kept focusing on the only way we'd have a good outcome: I needed to see warm and pink fingertips. After hours of hanging around the hospital and checking and rechecking his finger color, I headed home. Fatigue blocked all my emotions.

Driving home without listening to NPR on my car radio, I reflected on my experience. For the first time I could recall, the surgery held my attention without a typical mental intrusion from the outside. At a slow moment during routine surgeries, I usually have brief thoughts ricochet in my mind: *Stop on the way home for gas. Return a phone call. Check with Mary.*

In my absence Dr. Harrington checked the warmth and color of the patient's fingers every hour. Sleep eluded me that Monday night. After sleeping fitfully for three hours, I slipped out of bed without waking Mary and went to the hospital to check for dark fingers.

Returning him to microscopic surgery Tuesday would have been akin to competing in a Super Bowl game for two days in a row. We returned him to surgery on Wednesday. I held my breath as we gently unwrapped his hand. A throbbing pulse without leakage of the repair greeted us. The four original sutures held in both the artery and vein. Again, we squeezed the blood out of his arm and inflated the tourniquet. We began the second surgery with the experience from forty-eight hours earlier. I obtained rigid fixation with a plate and screws across the second wrist bone, the ulna.

Hallelujah.

When I'd adjusted his hand to work at different angles, two microscopic sutures had torn through the walls of the artery but not the vein.

More hours passed. We removed and replaced the two torn sutures of the artery and turned our attention to the nerves, also repaired while looking through the microscope. Throughout the procedures, we continued to drip normal saline onto the field to wash blood away and followed with miniature sponges to remove excess fluids.

In addition to the artery and vein, over a dozen tendons, muscles, and nerves passed through the top and bottom of his wrist. All had been severed. On the palm side, tendons bend the wrist and the fingers. On the back-side of a hand, tendons extend the fingers. The saw cut all muscles, tendons, and nerves at the same level. If I pulled every tendon together end-to-end, he would have a swollen mass around his wrist like a tourniquet. I elected to repair only the critical tendons first, the nerves last.

We rested after five hours of looking through a microscope.

Extensive therapy lay ahead for my patient, and more surgeries. I needed to build a team to join me in the challenge. No matter how exhausted I felt, I relished stepping into new territory in my operating room, knowing that the carpenter could have hope of eventually swinging a hammer again.

He healed without infection. With prolonged physical therapy for a year, he regained most of his range of motion, but his grip remained weak, sensation in his fingers decreased.

About six months after reattaching his wrist, another carpenter came in with a skill saw amputation of his right thumb. I reattached the thumb and his thumb survived with about 75% recovery.

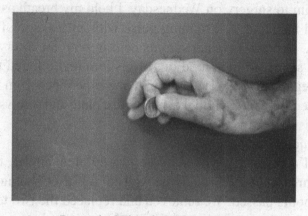

Reattached Thumb at Three Months

~~~

Until the 1980s no motivation existed for expediting hospital care. If not acutely sick or injured, patients were admitted for evaluation: lab exams one day, x-rays the next. Therefore, the patient may have lingered for days in the hospital out of convenience while the family discussed options. The hospital received Medicare payment for every day the patient stayed. Doctors reasoned no one knew what was better for patients than doctors, and we did so with arrogance. A patient with a repaired hip fracture was not pressed to roll from side to side, sit up, or learn to use a walker. We took a chest x-ray daily for pneumonia patients.

Despite resistance from physicians, Due to new rules, Medicare protocol changed regarding care and length of stay. Instead of paying for the procedure plus daily costs, Medicare began paying according to specific diagnoses or diagnosis-related groups. Thereafter, the hospital was paid once, based on the diagnosis, regardless of how long the patient was hospitalized. Insurance companies adopted the same rules.

Doctors and hospital staff stated patients could not be treated more quickly, but we learned the new protocol when reimbursement changed. We encouraged patients to move and learn earlier, decreasing hospital costs and complications. The longer a patient remained in bed, the higher the probability of a stroke, pneumonia, or infection. We listened more closely to lungs for progress instead of ordering x-rays. With reluctance, we learned to change.

~~~

During a routine surgery, I was driving a rod down a fractured femur of an elderly patient when it broke through the outside wall, creating a second fracture three inches below the first. Both fractures were clearly visible in the x-rays that glowed on the wall view-box.

My back and forehead broke out in a sweat. The normal level of low chatter ceased as the staff and I stared at the second fracture. Based on a risk-reward ratio, I had chosen to drive the rod down the middle of the femur as opposed to using a plate and screws. The patient had arrived in surgery with one fracture but now had two. The crew waited to see what I would do.

Every surgeon develops a profile regarding how he handles stress, surprises, or catastrophes. Some blame administration, equipment, or others. A few will curse and throw instruments. In all training programs, residents are exposed to a range of personalities. Although Monaghan raised his voice when he was stressed, he had provided advice over a beer one afternoon, saying I should rehearse how I would respond in a crisis, much like a fire drill. I had rehearsed.

"Thanks for helping me folks," I said to the staff and anesthesiologist. "I need to think about this." I stepped back from the surgery table and sat on a stool in silence.

Don't make a hasty decision I thought. The patient is stable. Look at my options. The resident is watching how I handle this.

I could remove the rod and make an eight-inch incision on his thigh long enough to expose both fractures and apply a plate with multiple screws. Perhaps I could pull the rod back and drive it on down across both fractures. If I removed the rod and applied a plate, and because his thigh was already open, I could also harvest bone from his pelvis for grafting. I elected to drive the rod across both fractures. I would not open his thigh for a bone graft. Each option carried advantages and disadvantages.

Although no one in the operating arena talked, I could feel them rooting for me.

I stood and returned to the table. "With your help, I'm going to pull the rod back and fish it across both fractures using x-ray."

To prevent collapse of the bone fragments, I placed a transverse-locking screw across the bone and rod at the top and bottom. When the x-ray tech hung the final films, they looked good. The rod fished through multiple fractures like a shish kabob, and the circulating nurse clapped for the team.

~~~

My career as an orthopedic surgeon has been sprinkled with bazaar cases and peculiar personalities who have shown up in the ER or my office. I imagine that many of these patients enjoy retelling their personal medical incidents every year at Thanksgiving dinners and family reunions.

In one case I handled, a good old boy had stopped at his favorite watering hole on his way home from work. After several hours, multiple beers, pool games, and stories retold, he left his buddies to return to his pickup truck where his other buddy, Sport, a Chihuahua, waited patiently for his master.

With careful planning and logic, he had tweaked his security strategy. Using the cup holder between the seats, he wedged the butt of his Ruger .22 automatic pistol pointing forward, like a cannon on a tank. He figured for a quick response to peril he could grab his pistol without looking, and it would already be pointed toward the threat. He could save seconds by not having to fish for his gun in a holster.

That night, before he could buckle the seatbelt, his excited companion leapt to welcome him back. Pushing off to leap into his master's arms, Sport passed his foot through the trigger guard striking the trigger and loosening the gun from its wedged position. Bam! The small-caliber bullet struck Walter's right fourth toe. The blast inside the truck and his master's yell frightened Sport. Trying to shake his leg loose from inside the trigger guard, the dog struck the trigger again. The second bullet shot out Walter's radio.

Gun smoke filled the cab. Walter's ears rang. Sport clawed at the passenger window.

Because the gun was small caliber and the bullet hadn't struck a vital area, Walter was able to limp back into the bar, leaving a trail of blood in his wake as he cussed and spewed.

"What the hell happened?" said one of his drinking buddies in the bar.

Silence fell as heads turned waiting for an answer.

"My dog shot me."

~~~

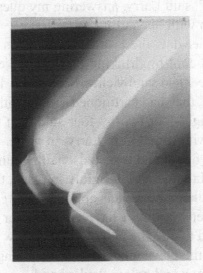

Side View of Nail in Knee

Most people wouldn't think that the profession of orthopedics involves a lot of carpentry, but it does. On a July day, I was finishing my office morning patients when an orthopedic resident brought me an x-ray of a finger nailed to a board. I proceeded to check it out.

Two men sat side by side in the ER, one a middle-aged man named Larry and the other his brother Paul, who was holding a beer in one hand and cradling a chunk of wood in his lap with the other.

As I looked closer, I realized Paul's right middle finger was nailed to two short blocks of two-by-fours in his lap. A leather glove had been cut away leaving a narrow strip wedged between his finger and the wood. The nail had gone through the glove, a finger, and a bone, but missed the cigarette stain between his index finger and middle finger. With enough beer on board, both men thought they were clever.

"I nailed my little brother to the wall," Larry repeated, his face shining as if this was an accomplishment.

They continued to interrupt each other during their story, pointing out the cooler of beer they'd brought to the ER.

Puzzled, I looked at the cooler.

"We didn't know how long we'd have to wait and it would get hot sitting in the truck." said Larry, answering my question before I could ask. He rambled on with his narrative.

On a hot summer day, the brothers worked as carpenters framing a house and stayed cool by drinking beer. They kept the Igloo cooler stocked with Bud beer and sandwiches. Seeing how fast they could work before quitting time, they had partitioned a room with two-by-four studs. Paul had held an eight-foot two-by-four stud next to another as Larry secured the studs with a nail gun. Larry, in haste, shot a nail through Paul's right middle finger and two studs, nailing him to the wall.

With Paul's right hand nailed rigidly in place, the brothers opened another beer and talked about their options. They explored the idea of cutting off his finger but didn't have enough beer to act as the anesthetic. Larry offered to pull the nail out with a claw hammer, but it was too buried to slide the claws under the head. Using a skill saw, Larry cut off the studs above and below Paul's hand.

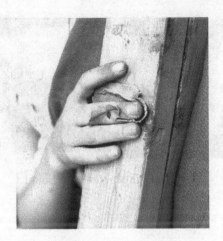

Finger Nailes to Board

Both men looked over thirty years old, but Larry was the oldest and dominant member of the duo. He spoke for both of them and carried at least forty pounds over his younger brother, filling out his Roundhouse bib overalls with a belly so big the shoulder straps pinched into his shoulders. Paul's bib hung limp with three pencils and a pack of cigarettes protruding from the chest pockets. The overalls on both brothers had the traditional hammer holder strap on the right thigh.

"Brother, I'm so sorry about that nail. It was all my fault, getting in a hurry," Larry said in a soft voice with his head down.

"It's okay," Paul said. "Love ya, brother."

"Want another beer?" Larry said to his brother, as though offering a beer in exchange for forgiveness. Paul turned and looked at me with raised brows.

"Not your best idea," I said.

X-rays from the front and side views revealed the nail to be perfectly placed through the middle finger. With Paul in surgery under anesthesia, I cut off the head of the nail with a bolt cutter. I rotated the blocks of wood back and forth pulling the nail on through, decreasing the amount of nail to be dragged back through the bone.

Paul's finger healed with good function, and I saved the strange x-rays, without a name or date, for my private file.

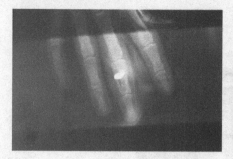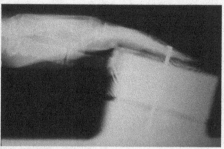

X-Ray of Finger Nailed to Board

~~~

Another carpentry victim showed up in the ER. The older man rested on the exam table with his knee bent. His grown son stroked his shoulder. The man's pant leg had been cut away and he had a small skin wound, no bigger than a pencil eraser on the outside of his knee.

I hung the front and side view x-rays on the view box. The front view showed the nail to be straight, but the side view revealed the ninety-degree bend of a big nail across his knee.

"What size nail is this?" I said, after introducing myself and trying to act as though I saw a nail buried in a knee every day.

"Four inches." He paused. "I'm glad it was the last damn nail in the clip. The clip holds twelve. I might have shot myself more than once."

His tongue thick from IV pain meds, the carpenter explained he had bee n standing on a three-foot-high scaffold using a new nail gun. Holding the heavy gun in his right hand over his head, he dropped his right arm to his side from fatigue and took a small step back. His right heel catching on a scrap of two-by-four, he lost his balance and fell backward. Grabbing for air with his left hand, he accidentally squeezed the trigger in his right hand. He shot himself above his right knee.

The four-inch nail entered above his knee, traveled through his fe-mur, crossed the joint, and entered his tibia. The gun had the power to drive the nail across two major bones up to the nail head. He fell three feet from the scaffold to the ground. When he drove the nail across the joint he was standing, but when he landed on his right leg, he bent his knee and the nail ninety degrees.

"I'll have to get the nail out," I said, stymied by the whole occurrence. "Surgery rooms are tied up for at least two hours. When did you eat last? I need your stomach as empty as possible."

"Breakfast at five-thirty this morning." It was now after eleven.

"Don't eat or drink anything. We'll be giving you more pain meds and antibiotics."

His stomach needed to be as empty as possible in case he vomited and sucked a piece of food into his lung. The anesthesiologist would determine which to give, a general or spinal anesthesia. If food was still suspected to be in his stomach, a spinal anesthetic would probably be used.

The carpenter's adult son continued to pat his father's shoulder.

While telling him the truth regarding how long it would be before surgery, I was also stalling. I had no idea how to remove the nail without damaging his knee. In about half an hour I planned take the x-rays to a scheduled lunch conference of orthopedic surgeons and get some ideas.

At lunch the other surgeons were equally as stymied.

"I have no idea," said one.

"It'll take at least two incisions," volunteered another. "Make an incision into the joint and cut the nail with some dikes or a bolt cutter. Bend the knee more, and pull out the lower half of the nail from the tibia. Since there's no head, you'll need a vise-grip. You can then pound the femoral part backwards. You'll need a second incision over the nail head and pull out the head with a claw hammer."

"Any way you do it will cause some damage to his knee," said a third. "Just because we can see it on an x-ray doesn't mean you can get to it. It's buried."

We quietly chewed our food.

"Straighten his knee with the nail inside," called a second-year resident sitting by himself at a back table.

We turned to listen to him, but another surgeon began talking. "If the nail doesn't straighten when you extend the knee, it will tear through the bone either above or below his knee," he said with a condescending tone. "You'll be worse off than ever with the busted pieces of bone in his knee and you'll still have a bent nail buried in one of the bones."

The resident looked around for a receptive face. "If the bone didn't tear out when it bent the nail, it shows the bone is stronger than the nail."

No one said anything.

He continued. "You can straighten the knee a little and check under fluoroscope to see if the nail is breaking through bone. If not, straighten a bit more and check again."

I went to surgery without a firm plan, but the resident's idea kept nudging at the edge of my thoughts.

I sent a request to maintenance for a carpenter's claw hammer. Although I had used wooden-handled hammers, I had never felt comfortable with the sterilization process. Even though they had been through the high temperature protocol, we wrapped them with sterile towels.

The carpenter rested on his back under general anesthesia, his right knee still bent to ninety degrees. At the risk of the bent nail breaking through the tibia or femur, I took a deep breath, supported his heel in my right hand, and began pressing down on his knee, waiting to hear or feel a sinking crunch. Not wanting my hands to be exposed to x-rays, I stopped pushing and checked the status of bone on both sides of the joint with the fluoroscope. I didn't see any injury to either bone, but the nail was a bit straighter. In ten-degree increments, I straightened his knee, stopping to check the status of the bone with the fluoroscope. I gained complete extension of his knee and the nail was straight in both side and front view.

Using the entry wound as a reference, I made a one-inch incision and exposed the nail head on the side of his knee that was buried flush with the bone. I teased a one-fourth-inch chisel under the edge of the nail head, creating space for the claws of the hammer. A sterile towel folded four times padded his skin and muscles and served as a fulcrum for the hammer's head. I eased the straightened nail from off the bone and rolled it in my fingers before passing it around the surgery crew.

"That nail is straight enough to be used again," said the scrub nurse.

Three stitches closed the incision and we were done in less than fifteen minutes.

"Success because of your idea," I said across the table to the second-year resident loud enough for all to hear, holding up the nail as evidence. I was glad he'd had the confidence to voice his unconventional idea amidst a group of experienced surgeons. Although he was wearing a mask, I knew he grinned because I saw the crinkle at the edges of his eyes.

~~~

I was coming out of the operating room after completing a routine surgery when the chief resident pointed to a man lying on a gurney in the hall.

"We need to take this guy directly to surgery. He was shot through his hand and the bullet lodged in his thigh. He doesn't want to talk."

Although pain medicine had been administered, I explained to the patient the nature of his problem in lay terms, including the need for surgery. He stared at the ceiling without a response. No family or friends accompanied him. As he was a handsome young man about twenty years old, I wondered what story he was hiding. His pain limited my examination of his hand, but x-rays of the destroyed bones provided enough information to know he would have limited use of the hand forever.

The experienced surgery crew prepped and draped him while the anesthesiologist put him to sleep. As I sat down to examine the man's hand, a uniformed policeman entered the surgery suite.

"You can't come in here," the charge nurse said, stepping in front of him.

He stepped around her.

"Which one of you is the doctor in charge?"

The behemoth with a badge on his chest and gun on his hip had to duck under the surgery lights. He looked as wide across his eyes as I was across my shoulders. The surgery suite had experience with visitors, but none this intimidating.

"I am," I said.

He just killed our Catoosa sheriff." No one said a word. "Our sheriff got a call about a holdup in progress and walked in on him and his buddy."

The room remained still. An air filter hummed in the background. Fumbling for words, the nurse gestured at a stool in the corner. "Uh, you can stay, but you'll have to put on a mask, shoe covers, and a head cover."

He scowled. "This guy and the sheriff must have shot simultaneously. We think the sheriff's slug is in this guy. Find it!"

X-rays hanging on the view box showed a bullet in the patient's right thigh. His hand revealed a one-inch entry hole on the top and an exploding exit wound covering his palm. About half of the skin from his palm was gone. The bullet apparently left small flakes of lead behind as it blasted through his hand bones, exited, and buried into his thigh.

While I was exploring his hand, the orthopedic resident explored the hole on the front of his thigh and searched for an exit wound. How were we to determine if the bullet that had passed through his hand was the same one still lodged in his thigh?

For grossly contaminated wounds such as these, we used a surgical power washer, which pumped out a pulsating stream of sterile saline. Turning his hand repeatedly palm up and down, I pumped liters of fluid into the wound from multiple directions. With a second washer, the resident irrigated the bullet wound in his thigh.

"Doc, I want that slug," said the policeman looking at the bullet in the x-ray hanging on the wall.

I temporarily abandoned the patient's hand and moved to his thigh. Using the bullet image on the x-rays as a reference, I slipped my finger through the apparent entry hole into the thigh toward the bullet. Because finding and retrieving a foreign body with my finger was highly improbable, I opened the wound one inch on each side of the entry hole with a scalpel, allowing room for retractors. I needed to see the status of the muscle along the bullet track.

The entry track looked like a hole that had been shot into mud. The mouth of the hole spread like a ragged funnel and the speed of the bullet had killed muscle along the walls. Pulling back the muscles, I could see

110

halfway to the bone. With dissecting scissors, I gently spread muscle tissue in line with the fibers. Usually I would snip away any questionable dead muscle as I went deeper, but in this instance, I had a different priority. I needed the bullet, and I knew I could trim the macerated muscle later in the procedure.

Although I followed the track down to the femur, I could not locate the bullet. Adjusting the retractors to pull in different directions, I explored behind more damaged muscle but could not locate the bullet, which was so obvious on x-rays. Probing gently with my index finger, I struggled in vain to find it.

"Call x-ray," I said. "We need the C-arm."

Surgeons frequently searched for a foreign body using a live fluoroscope. The arm resembling a giant five-foot "C" would straddle the patient. The arm could be used to view from side to side, then rotated and viewed front to back as the surgeon guided large tweezers to grab the foreign body.

We covered the C-arm with sterile drapes and rolled it into position over the patient's leg to view it from front to back. When I activated the floor pedal to see the bullet on the screen, everyone in the room could easily see it next to the femur. As the resident lifted the young man's leg, we rotated the C arm to see from side to side. To minimize radiation exposure to our hands, I took quick still images. The resident and I wore the dreaded lead-lined aprons.

Despite repeated still views from different angles, I was unable to physically locate the bullet.

Returning to the front-to-back view, I guided an instrument into the wound toward the bullet to grab it. Using the fluoroscope, I still couldn't locate the villain, a common occurrence with foreign bodies.

"I need three spinal needles."

Using spinal needles three inches long as markers, I inserted each point down to the bullet area from different angles, triangulating for orientation. Within minutes I found the deformed bullet.

"Doc, I want you to cut an X on that slug and look at it real close." The policeman spoke with a voice of authority and intimidation. "You'll be called to testify it's your X mark and you are the one who took the bullet out of him. You need to dictate it in your record."

The nurse handed me a scalpel with a fresh blade. I made my "X" and dropped it in the policeman's small plastic bag. Bullet in hand, he left the room.

Months later, I was called to court exactly as the officer had explained. My testimony required less than five minutes to tell my story and confirm the mark was mine.

~~~

Considering myself a lifetime learner, I worked at improving not only my practice skills but my communication skills, and occasionally these lessons presented themselves in a far more intimate setting than was comfortable.

When Mary began experiencing abdominal discomfort, our family physician referred her for an MRI.

As a doctor, I was familiar with the anatomy, but not the interpretation of what was revealed. My experience had been limited to studies of the arms and legs, plus the spine. I had known the radiologists within the x-ray department for years, and several were good friends.

Because I was a staff physician, I was welcome in the viewing room where the films were viewed and a report was dictated accordingly. The third year radiologist resident pulled up Mary's films on the screen. What he had to say became a defining event in my work.

I know what he said, but what I heard was that he was impressed with himself. He talked down to me in radiology terms I did not understand. A monologue that could have taken thirty seconds extended for minutes. When he slowed to take a breath, I realized I hadn't understood any of his report, and when he'd finished, I didn't understand any more than when I'd walked in the room. With Mary's history of cancer, I was concerned. I stood up and walked to another room where a staff radiologist was dictating.

"Can you pull up Mary's MRI?" I said.

"Sure."

He keyed her name and ID number, and multiple views of Mary's insides popped up across the screen. Within seconds he scanned her films.

"Can you tell me what you see?"

"I don't see anything bad, certainly no cancer. I do see some diverticulitis. Looks like it has probably been there for years."

I let out a breath I did not recognize I was holding.

"What to do about it is out of my line, but usually it responds to medication. Your family doctor will know." With apparent new awareness he looked me in my eyes as if finally comprehending the depth of my fear. "Mary is going to be around for a long time."

At a new level I understood why patients frequently appeared confused when I'd explained a medical problem. From that time forward, it became part of my job to check a patient's or family member's comprehension when I had explained the results of a procedure or a diagnosis. At that moment standing next to the staff member in radiology, I had to think of Monaghan's question that he posed so often after our Thursday lunches. *I know what I said. What did you hear?*

I sat on the same rolling stool in my office and listened to the same stories year after year, but I began hearing more. I no longer popped off the stool and strode to the x-ray box, speaking in medical jargon. Instead, I stayed in one place and listened more closely—hearing more clearly. When visiting with a patient I learned to monitor my choice of words regarding medical terms, including x-ray and lab results. Lay terms are less likely to be misunderstood. However, if the news was bad, I found it always best to address test results immediately in clear terms that were easy to understand. I never used the term "bad news" because the patient and family heard little of what more I had to say. Within the ever-changing scheme of cultural shifts and thousands of interactions with patients, two grown daughters, six grandchildren, I became a better listener.

I learned to listen to human suffering human in a different way, hearing a patient's pain with a deeper understanding. Repeatedly, I was surprised at how people and their families experienced, understood, and explained the same disease differently. In Malcolm Gladwell's book,

Outliers, he uses the 10,000-hour rule: "…you need to have focused practiced in your field of work 10,000 hours before you are good."

I also understood the rule applied to listening.

I attended a lecture at a state convention where the speaker stated that according to one study on listening, the average doctor interrupts a patient who is speaking within eighteen seconds.

Leaning in eyeball-to-eyeball, knees-to-knees and listening ever so closely, I gave my patients permission to pull all my energy. It felt good. At the end of an office day, I was often more tired than after a full day of standing in surgery.

Listen, Harold, listen, I kept telling myself.

Reading about pain and intellectualizing about illness was different from being in the presence of pain, illness, and *fear*. I don't recall a single textbook in my medical schooling that addressed fear or anxiety. Patients told me where and how much they hurt, but rare was the patient who admitted to being afraid of dependency, or job loss, or misunderstanding from others who could not understand how much they hurt. Despite their avoidance of these topics, I knew the underlying fear or anxiety needed to be addressed. The more I listened with focused intent, the clearer the stories unfolded and the better I could assist someone in facing those fears.

Because of my new appreciation of straightforward communications with patients, I wanted to slip learning incidents into the conversations with residents without being preachy—a fine line. I wanted to pass on important lessons in communicating with patients and their families, but I wondered if I might be getting too full of myself. Perhaps I was stepping into issues beyond my duty. Then I'd remember Monaghan who would not have taken time to clear his throat before looking me in the eye and addressing the lesson. I always envied his ability to address an issue head-on.

CHAPTER 6

ORTHOPEDIC PRACTICE

Tulsa, Oklahoma

1988-2010

I worked with an orthopedic nurse named Sherry for three decades. Together, we experienced the evolution of instruments. When a new one came to market, she wrapped and stored the outdated instruments. Because she stored them, only she knew where to find them. Perhaps it was a form of job security.

In general, most new surgery nurses shied away from orthopedics because of the need to gain expertise with a greater inventory of instruments, which required frequent additions. Within a decade, orthopedic instruments that once could be stored in a couple of drawers eventually needed a room of cabinets numbered by decade. By looking at a printed schedule the day before surgery, the surgical staff knew the instruments needed for a case.

In my third decade of practice, I stood scrubbing my hands at the sink with an orthopedic resident between Sherry and me. Feeling the need to break the silence and throw out some history for the resident, I said, "I can remember when we sterilized brushes and used them over and over. Now we use them once and throw them away."

"I can remember when surgery drapes were cloth and we did the same thing. Washed them, sterilized them, and used them for years," Sherry said as in a challenge to remember more.

Although we were looking straight ahead, our conversation morphed into a game of one-upmanship for the resident's ears.

"I can remember when doctors and staff smoked in the dressing room and we could smell the smoke on their fresh scrub clothes," I said, satisfied she couldn't match my turn.

She slowly leaned back and spoke across the resident between us.

"I can remember when you used to have a butt."

~~~

Driving accidents account for many of the patients who end up in the ER for treatment, but occasionally an injured driver wasn't driving a typical form of transportation. In one particular case, a forklift operator missed a ramp in a glass plant warehouse, and the machine turned on its side, pinning the man's left leg beneath it. Five fellow employees lifted the corner of the forklift and dragged him out from underneath the heavy machine.

X-rays showed no fractures, but he had no pulse on the top of his foot where he should have had one, meaning there wasn't any blood flowing through the arteries or veins because of the crushed and swollen muscles.

Arms and legs have a non-elastic thin layer of strong tissue, about as thin as Kleenex, around muscles. The enveloped muscles become compartments. In this man's case, although he didn't break a bone, his foot was still in trouble. Since the forklift had crushed the muscles behind his leg and below his knee, the progressive swelling in the surrounding compartments were creating too much pressure to allow normal blood flow. If we didn't do something quickly, the muscles would die a painful death.

Treatment consists of allowing the muscles to expand through longitudinal incisions of the skin and the walls of the compartments, a procedure called a fasciotomy (cutting open the compartments). An incision may range from four to twelve inches long. When incised, the wall of muscle in a compartment under pressure may quickly balloon through the incisions.

In this man's case, I made incisions on each side of his shin, and then rechecked for a pulse on the top of his foot. Nothing. I extended the incision two inches on each end. Still no pulse.

I could feel a weak pulse on the top of his foot, but it still wasn't strong enough for adequate blood flow. It might improve, but there were no guarantees. Whether his foot survived would be determined in the next few minutes.

"We need a Doppler," I said without looking up.

A simple Doppler machine is like a stethoscope on steroids. When this tiny ultrasound is placed over an injured area, it can detect the sound of a pulse before one can be felt. If a weak pulse is present, it will be magnified and heard by everyone in the room. We held our collective breaths and strained to listen as the nurse moved the Doppler tip over the site.

Nothing.

I lifted his leg to ninety degrees in hopes of draining a bit more swelling. The tension in the room was palpable.

A weak swish, swish, swish, echoed through the room. I longed to act but I knew better. The sound slowly grew louder and the surgery crew watched me, waiting for directions. I looked at the clock. "We're going to stand here and wait for another five minutes."

At four and a half minutes I could feel a weak pulse for the first time, but I continued to hold the leg straight up. When I could feel a strong and regular pulse, we started taking turns holding and lowering his leg.

The return of the pulse was good news, but I was faced with two twelve-inch incisions on the side of his leg that were stretched two inches wide. When there was a large amount of swelling in the wound, it would normally not be closed right away. Instead, the process would be completed in stages, with the patient being returned to surgery for progressive closure as the swelling subsided. However, in this patient's case, that could mean more trips to the operating room and more anesthesia time.

The senior resident eyed the gaping wound. "How about we lace him up like a boot?"

I looked at him. "What do you have mind?"

"Use the skin stapler on each side like lace holes, like a boot. Run two long sutures tied together at the bottom through the staples. Every day as the swelling goes down, we tighten the laces—right in his room. No need for surgery."

I nodded, impressed by his ingenuity. "That would require sedation each time, but sure beats returning to surgery to do the same thing."

"I need the staple gun," I said to the circulating nurse as though it was my idea. I began placing the tip of a hemostat under each staple to allow room for the suture to pass underneath it. I tied together the ends of two strong sutures, passed them loosely through the lower staples and tied them at the top, just like a boot.

Over days I progressively tightened the lacing as the the resident had envisioned; the skin edges came together on the eighth day and I sent him home on crutches the next.

Three weeks later, he returned to light duties on crutches.

~~~

One quiet night in the ER, an orthopedic resident named Dr. Simpson was working in a treatment room on a woman who had dislocated her shoulder. Interrupting him, an intern who was observing the case motioned his head toward the door. "I hear a ruckus down the hall." The nurse looked at the intern and cocked her ear toward the door. "Yelling and crying aren't unusual in the ER, but that doesn't sound right."

When Dr. Simpson stepped out into the hall, he saw two nurses lying on the floor and another on her hands and knees, blood dripping from her nose and mouth. A fourth nurse with a blood-splattered face was trying to pull her body up using the desk as support. The two on the floor were crying. The one on her knees groaned and cussed.

He stood frozen with shock. Then he heard groaning around the corner and headed in that direction. Two doctors were sprawled on the floor, one unconscious and the other trying to pull himself on to a chair. Directly behind them stood five thugs.

When they saw Simpson's 6'3", 230-lb frame and the rage that filled his facial expression, they turned in unison and raced toward the door.

Later Simpson said, "They were far enough away from me to make it to the car. If I'd been two steps faster, I would've run my fist through a window or jerked off a bumper."

Someone on staff called the police as Dr. Simpson returned to the building and began helping the wounded, each retelling an account of the night's mayhem.

According to the victims, a member of the gang had been drinking, stole a motorcycle, crashed it, and broke his leg. A fellow gang member brought his buddy with a broken leg to the ER. Then he called his thug buddies and complained about having to wait too long while his buddy received treatment, not knowing that thug in the next room waited for x-rays of his leg to be developed before a doctor saw him.

In what appeared to be an alcohol, or drug-induced frenzy, the four buddies arrived and charged through the door, cursing and swinging. The result was a trail of injured nurses and doctors, all because they heard their friend wasn't being treated quickly enough.

The police arrived and tried to get the guy with the broken leg to supply the names of his buddies. He glared at the first policeman and spat on the floor. "F... you."

A second, much larger cop moved in. "I'm going to ask again who your friends were."

The man eyed him defiantly. "F.... you, too."

The policeman shrugged and turned to Simpson. "Doc, there are a bunch of your friends who need your help. They'll need whatever pain medicine you have on hand. If there's any left, I guess you could give it to this guy, that is if he remembers any names." The policeman smiled at the man. "Wouldn't want the pain medicine to confuse him. Besides, he's not going anywhere. Go help your friends."

Simpson glared at the man, nodded, and headed for the door.

"Wait."

Doctor Simpson turned slowly on a heel.

Wincing in pain the thug said, "I...I remember now."

The policeman gave a slight smile and pulled a small notebook from his pocket. "Of course you do."

The policeman's partner had moved into the hall to question the staff. "Would you recognize any of them?"

"I would," said a nurse with a swollen eye and split lip. She delivered a vivid description to the policeman. "And the one who hit Darlene acted like he'd hurt his knuckles."

The policeman nodded. "Good, maybe he needs treatment. Notify the other ERs that these guys might show up."

Meanwhile, Simpson took care of the man's broken tibia and applied a leg cast. The police had him shackled and in the back of a cruiser before the plaster had even dried. One of the nurses was on the phone and held her hand over the receiver. "Hey! I'm talking to an ER that says they have a guy with a broken metacarpal on his right hand. He fits our description."

"Tell them to stall him," the nearest policeman said, tucking his notepad in his pocket, "until we can get there." He turned to the nurse who'd witnessed Darlene's attack. "Would you go with me and identify this guy? I'll make sure he can't see you."

"Let's go," she said, holding an ice bag to her lip and eye.

After the nurse identified him, the police made a quick arrest and snagged another of the perpetrators with him, one with an outstanding warrant and the other fresh out of prison on parole.

~~~

"Dr. B, we got a guy down here who's been attacked by a water hose." The ER resident stifled a laugh. "I can take care of it, but you might want to see it."

I had some free time before my next surgery, and the intern's teaser had piqued my curiosity. After I arrived, the husband and wife began their story. The patient had constructed a self-service car wash in his neighborhood and had installed metal components onto the end of a garden hose. Between the flimsy design and force of water pressure, one side of the hose blew out when he tried to adjust the setting.

"That thing jumped out of my hand and began whipping back and forth so fast I couldn't grab it. It happened on the driver's side and trapped me between the wall and car, banging up everything within reach, including me." He pointed to bleeding cuts and abrasions on his forehead and cheek. "I got my feet tangled in that crazy hose and fell on my left wrist."

He leaned toward me. "It was beating the hell out of me and I couldn't get up 'cause my wrist was broke and my feet were tangled up in hose. My wife jumped out her side and ran around to mine. She tried to grab the whipping hose, but it was too fast. It broke her glasses and got in several licks on her too. Her feet got tangled up and she fell on me. While the two of us were fighting that hose, she saw a valve handle and turned it off at the wall. Just look at her!" She was bleeding from small cuts on both arms and the back of her head.

His voice dropped to a whisper. "That thing is evil, I'm telling you. And you should see my fender. It's got at least a dozen dents. Looks like someone took a hammer to it. The metal connector knocked out my left headlight." I raised my hand in a thoughtful gesture trying to stifle a grin. "It ain't funny, Doc."

I recaptured my best poker face as the resident and nurse ducked out of the room. I could hear them giggling in the hall.

His wife laughed. "Glenn, if I look anything like you do, it *is* funny. The whole thing is ridiculous. We let a water hose whip the hell out of us!"

"Maybe someday, but not right now." The corner of his mouth lifted ever so slightly as he suppressed a grin.

I placed a cast on his left wrist. We sedated both man and wife, injected local anesthesia, irrigated the wounds, sutured small lacerations, and applied fourteen small dressings between them.

~~~

I have had elderly patients known to be high risks for surgery die shortly after a fractured hip was pinned. Because of pain without the surgery, the patient could not be moved for nursing and toilet care when pneumonia was days away. If the same high-risk patient could be taken to surgery where the fracture was immobilized, the patient could be turned and change positions to prevent pneumonia.

During one such procedure, I'd made a five-inch incision on an elderly patient's hip when the anesthesiologist, Dr. Sturdevant, spoke up while eyeing the monitor. "She's having a heart attack."

"What do I need to do? I just made a big incision."

"How fast can you do the surgery?"

"A few minutes."

He calmly watched her monitor. "Get after it then."

Usually I would've drilled in a small wire to confirm the position for the placement of the final pin and plate. Then I would've checked the position of the wire under the fluoroscope and repositioned the pin, if needed. Once I was satisfied, I'd normally drill over the wires and insert the final large lag screw and plate with more screws from the plate to the bone.

This was no normal day. I drilled without the check technique, inserted the lag screw, attached the side plate with every other screw hole, and stapled the skin shut, completing the procedure in nine minutes.

Luck was with both the patient and me that day. The patient recovered from both the surgery and the heart attack without problems. She was using a walker in less than a week.

~~~

"Battenfield, is that you I hear?" A deep voice carried from the adjacent ER treatment room.

"Yes," I said, responding to the unfamiliar voice.

"Stick your head in when you're finished there." When I completed caring for my patient patient, I entered the next room to see who had called my name.

"You don't know who I am," he said without introduction. "I've got water on my knee and it's killing me."

Following a brief history, looking at his x-rays and examining his knee, I determined he needed to have his knee drained for relief. A knee produces only enough lubricant to cover the walls and has the consistency of three-in-one oil. However, if the walls are irritated, the body tries to lubricate the problem away. When talking with patients I use the analogy of an irritant in an eye where tears are trying to wash out the problem. A knee functions in a similar manner, but without a mechanism for drainage. A knee with excess fluid can only bend to fifteen degrees and pain occurs from the swelling.

Tapping on the inside of his kneecap, I could feel the fluid wave on the other side, like water in a balloon. When only a tender touch on his knee caused pain, I knew I needed to drain the pressure from his knee as soon as practical.

Because ER doctors do not penetrate a joint on a regular basis and are reluctant to do so, they welcomed my presence. In my field I injected and drained joints as a routine.

When the nurse laid out the supplies on a tray, the needle captured the patient's wide-open eyes and he became anxious.

"How long is that needle?" His high-pitched voice filled the room. "Let me see it. No, don't let me see it. Put me out first."

My experience told me that a rational explanation would not work with the man. The burly fellow's appearance was inconsistent with his fear of a needle. His chart said he weighed 234 pounds. I ordered a good dose of pain and anxiety-relieving Demerol. Waiting on the medication to work its magic, I filled out charts for about ten minutes.

I injected his knee using a local anesthetic, waited a few minutes, and drained his knee, without causing discomfort. I removed enough knee fluid to fill a coffee cup, which gave him immediate relief.

The big fellow spoke with unfocused eyes, high on narcotics, a thick tongue and relieved of pain. "I need to sit up, so I can see you and talk better." He rolled from lying on his back on the examining table to his side and propped up on his right elbow. "But I need to lie back down a minute. I'm getting dizzy. Doc, you don't remember me do you?"

"No, but help me out," I said, trying to place his face.

"You put my hand together after I blow'd it off."

"I don't remember. Tell me more."

"Right there." He said pointing to a scar on the palm and back of his left hand. After examining his hand, a foggy memory tried to enter my mind.

"You had a gun injury, didn't you?"

"Yeah, but I never told you the whole story."

"Well, why don't you tell me now? There's nobody here but me and you." I figured a good story was wanting to be told.

He pushed himself up again to sit with his feet hanging off the table and leaned closer, implying his story was for my ears only. "Pull up a stool, Doc." Ducking his head, he looked around the room, searching for hidden cameras or eavesdroppers. He took a deep breath and braced his hands on the edge of the table.

I didn't recognize him because he said the injury had occurred five years ago, when he was a teenager. With an additional fifty pounds and a full black beard he was a different person.

"I was seventeen and had a date to the prom," he said. "I had the hots for this girl for a long time and finally screwed up enough nerve to ask her to the prom, even though I didn't know how to dance." Raising back up on an elbow, he leaned closer. His voice dropped to a whisper. "I was so nervous I could hardly ring the doorbell. She wasn't quite ready, so her mother asked me in to have a seat." He stalled.

"I'd been plugged up for five days because I was so nervous," he said, pausing as though the memory caused him discomfort. "Doc, I had been dreading that night." He shook his head, remembering. "All of a sudden I needed to take a dump, right then," he said, emphasizing with his index finger. "I asked where the rest room was and her mother showed me the way. When I was done wiping, I reached back and flushed." Another long pause followed because of his narcotic-soaked brain. He shook his head as if he was reluctant to tell me what happened next. "That's when I saw a pistol on the back of the toilet. Her daddy was a deputy sheriff." He blinked his eyes as though clearing his thoughts. "I couldn't leave it alone."

I waited to hear more.

"I picked it up. My pants were still down around my ankles. He stopped and closed his eyes, apparently retreating into a memory.

I waited. He took a deep breath.

"You ever been in a little biddy room when a big gun goes off? I don't remember pulling the trigger, but I shot myself in my left hand. I know I was done poopin' but my bowels opened up. It came out of me like lava and I stacked it up above the water line. I swear I felt like I sloughed three feet of my colon."

I didn't know whether to laugh or cry, so I settled on my best poker face.

"When her mom came runnin' in, I was screamin', shittin', jumpin' up and down, and turnin' and swingin' my arms all over the place. The room was full of smoke and I tried to run with my pants down, but all I managed to do was sling shit and blood everywhere—includin' all over the room and her and me!"

He leaned in closer to my face, his eyes wide. "She couldn't figure where the blood was comin' from. I was screamin' and she must have been screamin' cause I could see her mouth open and movin' cept I couldn't hear a thing cause of the roarin' in my ears. I knew I was hurt, but didn't know where. My date came runnin' in, saw all the commotion and started screamin' herself. And," he paused and shook his head, "you wouldn't believe what I did to her prom dress."

I leaned against the table and put my face in the crook of my arm. My shoulders began to shake.

When he caught me laughing he reached out, took my face in his hands and pulled me nose to nose. He frowned as he tried to focus, and his thick tongue slurred his speech. "Doc, it wasn't funny. It was horrible."

He eased down onto his back and let out a big sigh as he gazed at the ceiling.

"Well, you know the rest. You put my hand back on that night. Shootin' myself hurt less than thinkin' about gettin' out on the dance floor. Even now if I had the choice between shootin' myself or gettin' out on the dance floor, I'd shoot myself every time."

He missed the prom because he was in surgery. By simple luck the bullet had entered his left palm between two bones, nerves and arteries and exited on the backside, all without striking major anatomy. I had not put his hand back on, but that was how he recalled his experience. Like many patients telling their story, it had become embellished over the years until the fabricated version became factual.

One of my patients was a threatening drunk. He cursed the nurses when I would not write prescriptions for more pain meds. Hospitalized for three days for an infection in his knee, he badgered the nurses around the clock, complaining about the poor care. Yelling and cursing he scared other patients and attempted to fondle the nurses.

I dreaded entering his room, but did so one morning with a resident and a nurse.

"I know a doctor in Oklahoma City that can take better care of me," he said, pushing strips of bacon into his mouth that was already full of scrambled eggs.

"How would you get there?" I said.

"I'd catch a bus," he said in a defiant tone.

"How much does a bus cost?"

"Forty dollars." He took a gulp of coffee and spit it back into his cup. "Can't drink three-day-old coffee!"

I pulled forty dollars out of my wallet and handed it to him. "I'll hold the elevator for you."

He stuffed a biscuit into his front pocket and pulled the blue liner from a small trash can. The liner was his luggage. Pulling on his only pants, he stood with his back to us as he stuffed two packs of Camels into the blue bag.

"I don't have a shirt," he said in a more mellow tone. "Can I have this gown?"

"It's our gift to you," said the nurse.

He walked on crutches as I accompanied him to the elevator and held open the door.

~~~

My work in orthopedics required me to repair broken bones and to cover open wounds with skin grafts. I worked with emotional detachment at these tasks, knowing I was improving the quality of my patients' lives. My orthopedic training had focused on repairing and restoring. Knowing I could make a difference in someone's life gave me purpose.

Some limbs just couldn't be saved, but elective amputations did not fit under my mission to "improve the quality of life." I worked diligently to conduct procedures of repair, knowing incisions would heal, but an amputation altered a life forever. A somber event.

A few amputations became common, such as toe amputations in the case of diabetes. But when an entire extremity was involved, the operating room grew quiet. Everyone moved in apparent slow motion. When I handed off an amputated limb, it was surreal.

We honored and mourned the loss. I came to understand that not all injuries were fixable, but I never learned to perform the procedure without losing a piece of myself in the process.

~~~

No one from the outside world was permitted in to the sacred surgical arena, so there was no one to appreciate the carpentry skills of an orthopedic surgeon. It would have been nice to occasionally have a bit of an audience for our surgery crew. I wished my mother and Mary could have seen me work, and my daughters. I wanted them all to be proud of me.

If my two daughters could never see me labor and sweat in my profession, I wanted them to work sweating with me in the yard, getting our fingernails dirty. I drew joy from teaching them to use garden tools and manicure a flowerbed, sharing with them the great satisfaction of doing something productive and lasting with their hands.

restoring. Knowing I could make a difference in someone's life gave me purpose.

Some limbs just couldn't be saved, but elective amputations did not render my mission to "improve the quality of life." I worked diligently to conduct procedures or repair. Knowing incisions would heal, but an amputation altered a life forever. A somber event.

A few amputations became common, such as toe amputations in the case of diabetes. But when an entire extremity was involved, the operating room grew quiet. Everyone moved in apparent slow motion. When I handed off an amputated limb, it was surreal.

We honored and mourned the loss. I came to understand that not all injuries were fixable, but I never learned to perform the procedure without losing a piece of myself in the process.

No one from the outside world was permitted in to the sacred surgical arena, so there was no one to appreciate the carpentry skills of an orthopedic surgeon. It would have been nice to occasionally have a bit of an audience for our surgery arena. I wished my mother and Mary could have seen me work, and my daughters. I wanted them all to be proud of me.

If my two daughters could never see me labor and sweat in my profession, I wanted them to work sweating with me in the yard, getting our fingernails dirty. I drew joy from teaching them to use a garden spade and manicure a flowerbed, sharing with them the great satisfaction of doing something productive and lasting with their hands.

CHAPTER 7

COLLECTED STORIES FROM THE ER

"Wayne died first, but Doc beat him to the grave."

D r. Finley, a lone practitioner in a small Oklahoma town, came into my office limping. He wore a cast boot on his left foot and his left arm was in a sling. His wife helped him along by supporting his right elbow. With a thick tongue and speech slurred from pain meds, he gave me a history of his injury.

One week earlier he had served as a pallbearer for a friend in town, and he was assigned to be the middle pallbearer on the left side of the casket. After the funeral he helped load the casket into the hearse, which proceeded to the cemetery for the graveside service.

As the pallbearers had practiced with an empty casket the previous day, they pulled the casket containing his friend from the back of the hearse and began carrying it to the gravesite. A few of the mourners were wailing and some prayed out loud, but several buddies of the deceased, including a few pallbearers, had started the day by drinking. The lead pallbearer in front of Finley walked parallel to the end of the grave and turned left a bit too soon. Finley, who was looking to his right at the crowd, stepped straight into the six-foot grave.

Shocked, he reflexively tightened his grip on the casket's handle as he dropped out of sight, jerking the casket from grips of the other five pallbearers. It landed on top of his crumpled body. Pain shot through his right shoulder and left foot as the former dislocated and the latter broke. The casket stood almost vertical in the grave.

A woman screamed, mourners prayed ever louder, and a small pocket of inebriated old friends laughed out loud. Those on the front rows jumped up and gathered around the grave to see why Finley had disappeared. The other pallbearers tried to come to his aid, but they couldn't pull Doc out with the casket standing on top of him. Two young men from the crowd used the top of the casket to slide down into the grave to free him.

With the help of the pallbearers pulling and the two men in the grave pushing, they tugged the casket off Doc's foot. When they dragged the casket out they also moved it away from the grave. Finley was in too much pain to notice or use his injured right arm held tightly against his body. The two men boosted Finley from below and others pulled him out by his good arm.

Men from the crowd joined in pushing and pulling the casket until it was finally out of the grave. The funeral directors were aware that Wayne, the deceased, might be inside in a crunched heap. They carefully opened the casket to inspect Wayne—keeping their efforts from the family's view. They found him stiff and scrunched up toward the head of the casket, so they centered him again and combed his hair. A fluff here and a fluff there, and Wayne looked as good as…dead.

Some in the crowd cried, some laughed. The booze-laced crew tried to out-do one another: "They buried Wayne in a hurry," and "It's the fastest burial I've ever seen," and "Wayne died first, but Doc beat him to the grave."

Following heavy sedation, Finley's dislocated shoulder was realigned in the ER. X-rays showed a fracture of two small bones on the top of his foot. He wore a cast on his left foot for the fractures and cradled his arm in a sling.

One week after the injury, he told me his story in a serious tone. In attendance, his wife and daughter began laughing at the bizarre events and had to excuse themselves from the room.

I saw him three times in my office. The fractures healed and with physical therapy he made a full recovery with his shoulder.

My Anesthetic: Jim Beam

The sixty-one-year-old farmer had fallen off his roof while installing shingles. He came to the ER to have his dislocated hip fixed. The hip is a ball and cup joint and his fall drove the ball up and over the rim of the cup. Nothing was broken but the ball was painfully locked behind the cup. I pulled the ball back into the cup while he was under general anesthesia. X-rays revealed the weight-bearing top of his cup did not cover as much of his hip ball as did his left, an apparent congenital deformity. I advised him he may require a total hip replacement if the ball came out of joint again.

Two years later he returned with the same hip dislocated from a fall on the ice. Again, he did not break a bone, but the ball was out of place behind the cup. I pulled the ball back into the cup under general anesthesia. He completed a program of non-weight bearing with crutches and physical therapy. Again, I recommended a total hip replacement to prevent further problems. He would then be on crutches for several weeks. He declined the procedure because he was a farmer and could not take off work.

Two more years passed before he returned with a broken arm from a tractor accident. X-rays showed a non-displaced fracture of his radius above his wrist, requiring only a short arm cast.

"I haven't seen you in years," I said, applying his cast. "Did you ever have any more trouble with your hip?"

"We put it back in place," said his wife who sat in a corner chair.

"We?" I turned toward her. "Does that mean you helped him?"

"Every time," she said.

"When it came out of place a few years later, I figured you would give me some pain medicine and pull my leg back in place," the old farmer said, thumping his new arm cast that was almost dry. "I had an overhead beam with a pulley in my barn to haul hay up to my loft." He looked at his wife, pride shining in his eyes. "She helped me. We had a plan, so we didn't have to come back here where you put me to sleep and pull it back in place. You'd take me off work," he said shaking his head. "I couldn't do that."

"He couldn't do that," she said.

"When it came out of place, she hauled me to the barn in an old rusty child's wagon, then went to the house to get Jim."

"Jim?"

"Jim Beam. My anesthetic. We saved a bunch of money." He smiled. "I took three slugs of whiskey and made a loop for my ankle. I waited for the whiskey to kick in. I was on my back and we both pulled on that rope until my ass hung off the ground about a foot."

"Then what?"

"I took another gulp of whiskey and just hung there. After a spell, I wiggled my ass around and felt it go back in." He beamed with satisfaction and pride.

"Did it hurt?" I shook my head.

"Oh yeah. It hurt like hell, but I didn't have doctor bills or hospital bills and didn't miss any work on my farm."

"Has this happened more than once?"

"Yeah, three or four times. But I keep a rope hanging in my barn, plus one in my shop." As an afterthought he added, "I carry a rope and pulley in my pickup."

"A rope and pulley in his pickup," his wife said.

~~~

The Cowboy's Retirement

Patients appeared in the ER from every walk in life, introducing me to an array of interesting characters from diverse occupations. One such patient was a 53-year-old rodeo rider. This cowboy had been interested in buying a horse with a reputation for stopping quickly. Being able to stop fast was highly valued for chasing and roping a calf, allowing the cowboy to dismount, tie the legs together, and throw both hands in the air, stopping the clock. Calf roping, the horse and rider racing against the clock, was a popular competition event in a rodeo.

The potential new owner wanted to test the horse's stopping ability. The gate opened and the calf exploded from the shoot, running at top speed. His new horse leaped forward closing in on the calf. With years of experience and practice, he threw the rope around the calf's neck and cinched the rope on his end around the saddle horn, all within seconds. The experienced horse recognized the roped calf and stopped so quickly the rider's pelvis separated on the saddle.

"His pelvis broke open like a taco," said an orthopedic resident standing next to me as we marveled at his strange x-ray injury. His brief comment described the injury better than a lengthy x-ray report.

In males the pelvic bones come together in the front of the body with a false joint and are held together with ligaments one inch above the penis.

I'd never heard or read of such an injury and could not find a reference in any medical book. I took him to surgery and pulled together the one and half-inch separation between his pelvic bones. I used a small plate to bridge the gap and held the bones in place with two screws on each side. The following morning, two residents and a nurse accompanied me on rounds.

"Good morning," I said to the calf roper. "How did you rest last night?"

"Pretty good. I just took one pain pill," he said, consistent with being a tough cowboy.

"Okay if we look at your dressing?"

"Sure, that's your job."

I pulled down his covers.

"Oh my," said the female nurse. She took a step back, and the two residents joined her.

Overnight, the effect of gravity caused the swelling from his injury to drain into his scrotum. He lay with his legs apart, straddling his swollen scrotum resting on the bed. It resembled a water balloon ready to burst, the size of the swelling between a soft ball and a soccer ball. In addition, the skin over his scrotum had turned a brilliant, cobalt blue. As long as he didn't move, he experienced minimal pain.

We stood slack-jawed. Everyone waited for me to say something.

"Doctor, is it cold in here or is it just me?" he said, breaking the tension with a solemn face.

The swelling came from the surgery I'd performed above the site, and consisted of fluid within the tissues. Like water in a sponge, it couldn't be drained. The blue coloring resulted from bruising that had settled in his scrotum. When I examined the scrotal skin, it still retained elasticity and only appeared to be tight.

"Doc, it doesn't hurt until I try to stand up. Then it's a real problem."

He could not urinate while on his back, but the weight of his scrotum was too painful to stand. Few men can urinate without their feet on the floor, whether standing or sitting. He needed support, somewhat like an arm sling.

We cut and fashioned a giant sling from a sheet and passed it under his scrotum and tied it around his neck. To support his scrotum and relieve the weight on his neck, he leaned his head back to distribute some of the weight of the sling across his chest. He stood and walked leaning back while looking at the ceiling. Using a walker to relieve weight on his injured pelvis required him to apply weight on his hands. Therefore, his hands were free to cradle and relieve the weight on his scrotum. The nurse led to him to the toilet. He was unable to sit and urinate because with the size of his scrotum, there was no room in the toilet for it to fit. Therefore, he was confined to standing to urinate while looking at the ceiling. Even his neck grew tired from supporting his swollen scrotum.

Medication or further surgery wasn't indicated, but we elevated the foot of his bed and applied ice packs. The swelling subsided enough by the third day to release him for home.

Hospital personnel delivered him in a wheelchair to the exit door, but he needed the walker for the last few steps to his car. When he walked, he did so looking at the sky, which attracted curious onlookers.

Two weeks later, he returned to my office using one crutch.

His wife shook her head. "I walk in front of him because he embarrasses me. He uses that crutch with one hand and, when he comes to a curb, he grabs his crotch and lifts it with his other hand."

The cowboy healed well, but he gave up competition rodeo.

~~~

A Captive Audience

Patients are human beings with human emotions that can't always be controlled, as I discovered with a sixty-six-year-old woman I treated. She had fallen on a throw rug, bruising her left shoulder as well as breaking the skin of her elbow and left knee. She had been kept in the hospital for two days for evaluation of other potential injuries.

I stood by her bed. "Your x-rays look good with no breaks. I am going to dismiss you in the morning." She nodded.

The following morning, I entered her room with her chart.

"I don't feel like going home today," she said.

"Are you in pain?"

"I still have bruises and feel sore all over."

"I see on your chart that you haven't taken any pain meds."

"Sounds right."

"Do you have a problem at home that I need to know about?"

"No."

"Then why don't you want to go home?"

"I live alone and get lonesome." Her voice quivered. "Medicare pays my hospital bills and insurance covers the rest."

"How long are you expecting to stay?"

"I haven't decided." She turned on her side, propping her head up with the heel of her hand.

Backing away from her bed, I wondered what action to take. I had never experienced such a dilemma. During lunch, I surveyed three colleagues at my table and came up with three solutions: hide strong laxatives in her food, put her on a low-calorie diet, turn on acid-rock music. They responded in jest because they had no practical suggestions.

The next morning, I dreaded seeing her more than caring for an injured drunk in the ER.

"I'm ready to go home after lunch," she said as soon as I walked in the door. I was simultaneously stunned and relieved.

"What made you decide to go home?"

"I couldn't get TV reception for my favorite soaps: *As the World Turns* and *All in the Family.*

135

~~~

A Bit of Magic in Medicine

A nine-year-old boy with a broken arm waited for me in the ER. X-rays revealed a forty-five-degree angulated break two inches above his right wrist. The bone needed to be set and casted. Because setting the bone would be painful I favored general anesthesia. However, the boy had just eaten two hot dogs. If a general anesthetic was administered with a full stomach, he could vomit and aspirate food into his lungs. Many hours needed to pass before the hot dogs were digested. Complicating the injury, the shock of trauma caused his body to slow digestion even further. No food or water provides time for the body to digest all food and safely administer a general anesthetic before setting a broken bone.

Providing heavy sedation along with a local anesthetic was also an option, but was a technique usually preferred for older, cooperating patients.

I showed the x-rays to the father and son and explained the safety of an empty stomach for general anesthesia and recommended returning in the morning.

"Let me talk to my son a few minutes," he said politely, moving between me and his son. I assumed they were going to pray about the matter.

"Certainly." I stepped back and waited.

The father stroked his son's arm ever so lightly. He spoke in a soft, slow, monotone voice. "Close your eyes," he murmured. "You're doing well. You're going into a deep sleep and the doctor is going to set your arm. You won't feel anything and when you wake your arm will feel normal."

My jaw dropped. I wanted a witness to what I was seeing.

His father nodded to me. "Okay doctor. Do what you're going to do. He's ready."

"Do you need anything?" said a nurse coming in to help me.

"Yeah, come on in here and watch this," I said.

With apprehension, I picked up his crooked arm and tested for pain by pressing my index finger over the fracture. Nothing.

I looked at the nurse in disbelief. She shrugged and nodded me on. We were witnesses to the power of hypnosis. I placed my thumbs over both sides of the fracture and, as if breaking a large stick, snapped the fracture into alignment. An x-ray tech rolled in a portable machine and snapped a front and side view, confirming the bones were well aligned. While the boy was still under hypnosis, I applied a full-arm molded cast, all without any sign of discomfort. Even with sedation and local anesthesia, a patient experiences some pain, but this case was different.

"I'd like to take it from here," said his father.

I laid the boy's casted arm across his abdomen and stepped back, not knowing what to expect.

"You did well, son," the father said continuing with a soft voice and stroking the boy's fingers protruding from the plaster. "You did well. When I count to three, you will open your eyes, feel no pain, and we'll go home." The father counted to three and snapped his fingers. The boy opened his eyes and blinked twice. Wanting to be more useful, I helped him sit up.

Still unsure of what I had witnessed, I waved my hand in front of his eyes as though I would expose the act. He blinked normally as if I were the one in question.

I handed the father written instructions with my phone number, and told him to return to my office for a follow-up visit.

When I sat to dictate, I stopped short of the memorized lines I had used hundreds of times to describe the routine setting of an arm. In all other cases, my dictation started with "Under general anesthesia..." or "Under sedation and local anesthesia..." Instead, I stammered, erasing and backing up the tape three times. Finally, I spit out what happened, "With my patient under hypnosis by his father, I performed..."

The Disobedient Patient

A small segment of my patient population could not, or would not, follow instructions. A sixteen-year-old boy came to the ER by ambulance with a severe, type three fracture of his left tibia. Between sobs of pain, he said he and his motorcycle slid across a road, through gravel, and in front of a car. Because the driver hit his brakes, the car's wheels were not turning, as one car wheel dragged over his left leg, it pulled away skin, muscle, and one side of his tibia.

During his surgery, I washed the wound and picked endless bits of gravel from his muscles, bones, and remaining skin. The treatment of that era for such a fracture was either the application of a plate with screws or external fixation. A plate was not indicated because the remaining skin was insufficient to cover it, so I settled on external fixation. I drilled transverse pins above and below the fracture and attached them with bars outside of the skin, somewhat like a scaffold on a building.

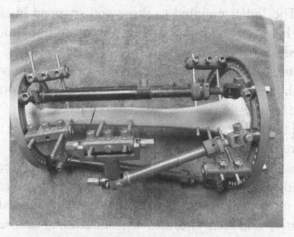

In external fixation only the pins penetrate the skin - temporarily used when there is a loss of skin and muscle

With multiple skin grafts over several months, the wound eventually closed, but the bone didn't heal. After a year of care and crutches, electrical bone stimulators entered the market. I ordered one and attached it to his leg. The patient plugged into an electrical wall outlet three times a day for thirty minutes. Months passed. Marginal healing could be seen on x-ray. I removed the external device and applied a non-weight-bearing cast.

He was instructed not to apply weight on that leg and always use crutches. Instead, he chose to ride behind a friend on a motorcycle and wrecked again—fracturing through the new bone growth that had been so carefully coddled. Regardless of the cast I applied, it never held up for long—since the bottom of a long leg cast would break down in about a month or six weeks, due to weight bearing and moisture.

The likable teenager stayed with me so long that I watched him mature and grow his first beard in the twelfth grade. When he came in for a cast change, he helped himself to the storage cabinets and had all the supplies gathered for me as I entered the room.

He graduated from high school with a full leg cast. One month later, I saw enough evidence of healing to remove the cast—with the agreement that he would be very cautious for the next several months and use a cane as a reminder.

He rode a motorcycle to my office for his final visit.

Out of Joint

"Do I see *both* shoulders out of joint on this x-ray?"

"You sure do," said the resident who was assisting me in the ER.

After dozens of years of experience, I expected to hear the story of a fall or car wreck in which someone used both arms to brace against the dashboard.

The sixty-year-old woman in the ER had both arms extended in the air above her shoulders. Her husband stood in front of her, holding her by her wrists. She could bend her elbows, but not her shoulders.

He explained that they had been attending a religious revival at Oral Roberts University and had responded to an altar call. With arms raised to praise the Lord, both of his wife's arms had locked when she flung them straight up in the air.

"It was a painful ride for her to the hospital, I tell you," he said.

"Where do you hurt?" I asked her.

"My shoulders are killing me. My elbows and hands are tired but okay." Her husband supported one arm while I examined the other. X-rays confirmed both shoulders were dislocated, which meant we would both have to manipulate and pull both back into their respective joints. I had never seen or even heard of this kind of shoulder dislocation in all my years.

Waiting for the pain medication to take effect, the orthopedic resident made a quick trip to the library and found a reference concerning a patient who was in an erect position when the shoulder was dislocated, and the reference included instructions for pulling the joint into a normal position again. Most shoulders presented in the ER were dislocated with the ball out of joint below the socket and the patients held their arms across their abdomens.

Following heavy sedation, I applied traction to her left arm and manipulated her shoulder back into its normal position. I did the same with the right shoulder. Repeat x-rays revealed both shoulders to be in good position and she left the ER with each arm in a sling.

The technical diagnosis was *luxation erecti*. Most orthopedic surgeons will never see one in their life; I treated two in the same night on the same patient.

I never saw another bilateral shoulder dislocation case or even heard about one.

Clowning Around

Working in the serious business of surgery and witnessing all kinds of human suffering in the ER would be overwhelming without humor to break the day-to-day tensions, and hospital staff never failed to take advantage of an opportunity for comic relief, especially if the joke was on me.

I had been working with a patient from a car accident until midnight, and early the next morning, I had a fractured femur to plate. The plate was straightforward enough that I allowed a senior resident and first assistant resident to gain needed experience. I needed rest.

In the surgery room I elected to sit in a chair wearing a lead apron like the residents. It hung around our necks like a kitchen apron, tied at our waists and extended to our knees, protecting us from radiation. Warm and idle, I fell asleep and rolled off my stool.

Awake before I hit the floor, I jumped up and looked around for witnesses. Quite apparently, there were none. I gowned again and entered the sterile field.

When I entered surgery the next morning, a lone chair sat in the corner with a shoulder strap over the back of the chair rest.

~~~

On another occasion I had been requested to consult on a patient hospitalized for a chest and pelvis injury, but I was to evaluate only his pelvic injury. As per my routine, I reviewed the patient's x-rays before the examination, enabling me to tell the patient more about my findings and recommendations. Two orthopedic residents accompanied me to the x-ray department to examine films of his pelvis.

"Here is a non-displaced fracture of his pelvis on the right side," I had said pointing to a crack in his pelvis. "If I press lightly here over the fracture, it'll be very tender." I explained the correlation of x-rays with clinical findings of local tenderness or pain when pressure was applied, even light pressure.

Shaking the patient's hand in room #405, I introduced myself to the man along with the residents, and explained they were in training and I would be discussing his case.

The fracture was in the pelvic bone located under the patient's scrotum on the right side.

"Is it okay if I examine you?"

"Okay."

"Please pull up your knees and spread your legs."

He did so by pulling up his hospital gown and spreading his legs. With gloved hands, I lifted and gently pulled his testicles to the left.

"He will be tender on his right side about right here," I said with authority to the residents. I applied slight pressure on his crotch with my thumb. "Is that tender?"

"No."

"How about here or here?"

"No....no."

Thinking I may have the wrong side, I lifted and moved his testicles to the right and applied pressure several places.

"Here...here...here?"

"No...no...no."

"That means the fracture is healing and stable, although I can still see evidence of the fracture on x-ray." I removed my gloves and shook his hand. "I recommend walking on crutches for a couple of weeks or until you can walk without hurting. You will heal well."

Out in the hall I elaborated to the residents that the patient's symptoms didn't match his x-ray, not unusual with pelvic fractures.

The following morning the two residents met me outside room #406.

"Yesterday we turned too soon into room #405." The senior resident could barely keep a straight face. "We examined the wrong guy. We should have gone one room further, room #406."

~~~

Once a month our department gathered in the evening at someone's home and selected an article to review from an orthopedic journal.

One night when the resident finished his review, we hauled out the beer sponsored by an orthopedic supply company.

Lee was recognized as the comedian of the group and held our attention. With minimum embellishment, he began exposing our personalities wrapped within a scenario. "If a fire broke out in a theater, Ed would jump up in the seat and yell, 'Fire! Fire! Let's get the hell out!'"

Everyone laughed because they agreed.

"Jeff would look up and down the aisle and turn back to the screen to watch the hero for a few more seconds."

Everyone laughed because they knew Jeff.

"Dr. B would say, 'Let me tell you about a fire I was in.'"

Everyone laughed. A stab to my heart could not have been more effective because Lee had told the truth. Until that experience, I did not realize that I was sometimes stealing another person's thunder, albeit without intending to do so. I smiled at Lee, grateful that his accurate humor had led me to an important truth about myself.

~~~

CHAPTER 8

RETIREMENT REFLECTIONS

Tulsa, Oklahoma

2010-2017

In all my years of practice, I had only two malpractice lawsuits filed against me. As one learns from their elders, I learned to be afraid of malpractice from my trainers and older staff members. I first heard the term when I was a student, as a threat that existed only in the future. As a resident in the lunchroom, I heard doctors talk about the injustice of frivolous claims against them. By the time I entered practice, the threat of malpractice was ingrained in me. I'd been exposed to the fear through nine years of education. The indoctrination was complete.

In most states, doctors qualified for a reduced rate on malpractice insurance if they attended a minimum of one course per year regarding how to avoid, handle, and undergo a malpractice claim. Conference speakers admitted that screws break, plates bend, and infections happen, but consistently the speakers pounded home that a poor doctor-patient relationship was the major factor in most malpractice cases. If the surgeon projected lack of concern for the patient, he was at a higher malpractice risk whether complications occurred or not.

We were coached not to focus on potential litigations because the surgeon could begin to perceive each patient as an adversary. But the public was also being indoctrinated through new television dramas. As television shows presented fantastic dramatizations of medical care, the public became more prone to form opinions about how medicine should be practiced, without having full knowledge of the intricacies involved.

In the interest of tidy one-hour shows, patients on TV dramas recovered in thirty to sixty minutes, and distortion of reality became the norm in the medical profession. If a villain or hero on television wanted to render someone unconscious for a few minutes, he could be lightly tapped on his head from behind with the butt of a gun, and to be "knocked out" longer required a stronger blow. Regardless of the power of impact, a blow to the head on television was treated as a temporary setback with full recovery occurring in minutes. If the hero of a movie needed to be wounded near the end of the story, he was shot in the shoulder or "winged," implying a shoulder wound was not serious, and it was usually healed by the next week's episode. In reality a bullet to a shoulder might not kill a person, but it would likely produce a permanent disability—something never shown on a TV drama.

One of my malpractice cases was instigated by a television advertisement. The ad called for anyone who'd had a catheter inserted to deliver local anesthetic for postoperative pain to join in the malpractice suit. Although I hadn't used the specific brand of catheter named in the settlement, I was caught in the broad net of a claim that lingered for years.

The other malpractice lawsuit resulted from a consultation in my office for a one-week-old fractured wrist in a cast. I recommended surgery with a plate and screws. The patient went on to have the surgery by another surgeon with a good outcome but claimed I should have made the recommendation earlier. I had only seen the patient once. My insurance settled the case as a nuisance, but because I'd been blindsided by the complaint, I questioned my competence and integrity.

Medical malpractice claims occur in the U.S. far more often than in other advanced countries. Medical litigation costs overall are at least twice those of other developed countries. Although most are frivolous, a malpractice case may linger for years, exacting a price. It is not unusual for the stress of a prolonged case to spill over into the home front, resulting in trouble and even divorce. The doctor may have to leave the community regardless of the outcome, especially if the practice is in a small town.

As a teaching aid and also for legal protection, I stored a camera in my locker and photographed certain cases. If I inherited a case from the ER with a predictably poor outcome, I had only one opportunity to document the severity of the injury before time wiped away all visual evidence of the initial trama. X-rays revealed only the status of bones, which may show them to be in good order, but the mangled soft tissue—muscles, nerves, or skin—would not show on an x-ray; nor could an operative report describe in pages of text what one photograph could demonstrate.

By definition of an emergency, the patient is traumatized, confused, and frequently intoxicated. The problem is often compounded by the presence of a frightened family. I photographed trauma cases, especially the ones that would be impossible to repair, only salvage. I took several photos various views, and I included with the images the patient's initials and date. A healed amputation with healthy skin covering the remaining bone might cause one to wonder why the surgeon would remove a foot, arm, or leg, and a dictated description in the operative report did not compare to a photograph of a mangled foot in living color.

I filed the photos in their respective patient charts, hoping never to need them. On four occasions the patient and family returned for follow-up in my office and questioned the outcome. The conversational tone bordered on hostility. On seeing the photos, the patient and family understood the extent of the injury and were satisfied with the care.

The camera was for, CYA—cover your ass.

~~~

In the decades following the Vietnam War, high school graduates interested in continuing their education could usually find a good college fit. Except for prestigious schools, colleges in general were straightforward and had limited competition for acceptance. However, to be accepted into medical school, the odds against an applicant could be discouraging. The percentage admitted fluctuated within the geographic location, era, and economy. When I graduated from medical school, only one in three applicants were chosen for a specialty. The progressive selection process generated unintended consequences of "I am special."

A medical diploma implied that power had been granted to the degree holder concerning a specific field in medicine, but it did not teach the new doctor to appreciate and use the power responsibly, and medical courses didn't address respectful use of power, either.

The power of easy financial credit became apparent as new cars began to sprinkle the parking lot. Unintentional power was issued in subtle ways to doctors: reserved parking in convenient spots, private dining rooms in hospitals, and no consequences for excessive delays in seeing patients. Patients might be kept waiting for hours to see a doctor, despite having a specific appointment time. When beginning practice, a new doctor understood the need to be on time, but as his practice stabilized, long lunches and overscheduling became the norm. Could such frequent and insidious considerations alter a doctor's self-importance and become a blind spot, resulting in an attitude of entitlement?

"My afternoon appointments started at 1:00," said one of my peers as we ate lunch. The wall clock over his left shoulder said 1:25.

"Mine too," added another peer.

Without calling attention to the clock, I proposed a casual survey at the lunch table by questioning if anyone could recall having to wait in a doctor's office an excessive length of time. All four at the table had experienced waiting on a doctor, and although they could recall only vaguely their medical problem and the name of the doctor, they remembered the waiting room in vivid detail, as well as the discomfort of sitting without information for an hour or longer. The experience was magnified if a patient was waiting on a MRI, x-rays or lab report that might carry a life-changing prognosis.

Multiple studies have revealed that a patient will wait for about thirty minutes on an appointment before resentment begins. After an hour the relationship is damaged, and the opportunity to develop a good relationship is compromised. The major complaint against a doctor is not high cost or poor listening skills but waiting, waiting, waiting.

Another factor contributing to a doctor's sense of privilege and power is the rating system ingrained in training programs for doctors. Beginning in college, I was ranked along with the other students, our grades sometimes posted on the bulletin board. Although ranking was not always posted, we learned of our general rank through the grapevine and coffee talk. Within a few days I knew how I'd scored on a recent exam by listening to hall chatter. In medical school, ranking was the absolute status symbol, and it continued through state board examinations. I carried an invisible number on my back like a tattoo.

When I began practicing, I displayed my diploma where patients could see it. After several years, I realized no one ever asked about my class rank, where I went to school, or if I even went to school. I could have left my diploma in a drawer at home; a simple print hanging on the wall picturing three ducks taking flight from the surface of a still lake would have been more interesting.

One day at lunch, I asked three of my colleagues, "Do you remember your medical school rank?"

"Yes," said the first, "Yeah" said the second, and the third one nodded in agreement with the first two.

"Has a patient ever asked you what it was?" I said. They shook their heads. "How about where you went to college or medical school?" I received the same response.

"Are you a good doctor?" asked Mike, sitting across from me. Before I could answer, he extended his question to the remaining two. We all agreed we were good doctors.

"Good is a relative term," Mike said looking around the table. "If we're all good, then someone has to be above average and some below." He paused long enough for us to process the point. "We all passed the state board examination to get a license. There's no valid way to rank us in practice.

"Who would set the bar, and at what level?" said Raymond. "We all get a new license every year. We have to document that we sat through continuing medical education classes to do it."

I pondered the issue and retreated to the adage, "Patients don't care how much you know, only know much you care." It made me wonder how we could measure how much we care. "Care is judged by clues. They want the doctor to be engaged and truthful, but they want to leave an office with hope. We all know we're going to die, but we hope for comfort, for happiness, and for meaning before we get there."

"I see it like professional pilots," said Mike. "There's no way to measure one against the other or rank them. They're all well trained, they all passed the exams, and they have to undergo continual training." He paused as though collecting his thoughts. "We're no different."

Old indoctrinated habits edged into my thoughts. Although Mike went to a different medical school, I wondered how he'd ranked. How did I rank in my class compared to him? Asking someone about their rank would be as inappropriate as asking about their sex life or bowel habits. Was I jealous or simply competitive, and if so, didn't this attitude grow out of my own indoctrination to medicine?

Would I ever outgrow such thoughts?

In pondering how I chose my own doctor, I realized it was not by his class rank but by how much he cared. I could identify that trait by observing a doctor in a short conversation: Does the doctor want to listen or talk? Does he seek to be engaged with or speak at his patients? Are his words obvious or oblique? Does he nod appropriately, showing he understands and empathizes?

While trying to listen to the rest of the conversation that had enthralled my colleagues, I silently chose Mike to be my doctor, not because of an imaginary class rank, but because I could tell he cared.

As I listened to the conversation, I understood Mike had made the transition into a caring doctor somewhere along the journey during his two decades of practice, but if I asked him to define his learned art he would fumble for an answer, and probably be embarrassed. Trying to define the art of caring is about as subjective as one can get. I tried not to say another word but to listen.

I realized that if I could be ranked as a doctor, I could also be ranked as a father or grandfather. If I had to rank success among important roles of my life, I would settle for being the best father or grandfather.

"Robert died," our senior partner Dr. Campion announced to me over the telephone on a Saturday in 1980. Dr. Peele had died at age fifty-two after smoking for nearly four decades. No signs or symptoms had warned him. As was common with smokers, his office ceiling was stained from nicotine. He died deeply in debt.

My father died that same year, and in the vacuum created by these two important men in my life, I found myself needing a mentor.

In 1982 our office recruited from our training program an orthopedic surgeon who had an additional fellowship in sports medicine. Dr. Nebergall had the body of a weight lifter and a captivating smile. He taught the residents to perform sport physicals and arranged to have a resident present at local Friday night football games. Our office started staying open on Saturday mornings for further care of Friday night injuries to young teenagers, some requiring surgery. I saw firsthand the ravages of Friday night football injuries to teenagers, and Dr. Nebergall championed these young people. Many former high school athletes would show up in our office decades later for knee replacements.

Dr. Nebergall died at age fifty-nine from alcohol-related illness. He had been divorced from his second wife, and he left behind a small child. I wanted a role model.

Dr. Bauer joined our staff following a fellowship in spine surgery. He had an amazing ability to identify patterns of practice and how to respond to unaddressed issues and needs. He projected directions our practice needed to investigate and explore. His intellect, however, did not filter out a love of motorcycles. The thrill of the wind took his life at age forty, and he'd been divorced with two children. His sixteen-year-old brother was killed on a motorcycle years earlier.

I wanted a role model—someone who went beyond expertise as a surgeon and strived for excellence in private life as well.

In 1996 Dr. Campion retired at age seventy-two with his third wife. Due to limited savings and two ex-wives, he elected to go to a trade school for heating and cooling. He built three houses before he died in 2006.

Throughout the years I realized three of my four partners died from preventable causes. The last orthopedic surgeon in my life who had lived a productive life with the same wife and affordable retirement was Monaghan. I had to reach back over forty years to find that simple combination.

The most dependable foundation for me in life was my stalwart Mary, and I built a stable life on that foundation. Along with family stability, I valued education. I discovered CD recordings of classes and motivational speakers, and I always had a CD ready to play in my car if I was alone. I love to learn. I played with numbers regarding lost time in a car and extrapolated if the average person drove 13,000 miles per year at the average speed of thirty miles per hour, one could derive the equivalent of a college education every five years just by listening to educational recordings during dead time in a car.

Until Dr. Campion retired, I had viewed myself as a young man entering practice. When I became the senior partner in our practice, it was my time to be the role model for others.

Where had the years gone? As an assistant or partner I had always looked to my senior partners for expertise. When I became senior partner I had more experience than my junior partners, but I needed to remind myself that I wasn't necessarily wiser. My two younger partners amazed me with their insights into complex issues and their ability to understand policy issues and long-term consequences. I also needed to remind myself that although I was the senior, I was not the boss, contrary to the way it had been when I entered the practice. If our personnel had a policy question, they had always waited to deal with it until Dr. Campion was in the office, and I had learned to do the same.

When my new younger partners and I sat in office meetings, I became aware of the percentage of time that I talked. To my surprise, when I focused on listening instead of talking, our meetings grew shorter and shorter. Nothing changed but my awareness regarding office policy and my responsibility to act with diplomacy. In the past our personnel were conditioned to bypass junior partners, but I wanted to change the office culture. If I needed to address concerns or staff problems with my partners, I discussed the issues in an office meeting, not in the halls where conversations could be overheard by others. As mentors in our practice we agreed to know the relevant details about the lives of our personnel and their children, just as we concerned ourselves with the welfare of our own families.

~~~

Sometimes I am asked if I miss practicing medicine. Pressed to give a valid response I condensed my answers to two points: I miss the orthopedic residents who were always curious and full of energy, and I miss our office staff that comprised a family team. I worked with some of them for decades and knew their children and watched them grow, making my own life fuller by appreciating theirs.

As my years in practice accumulated, the list of poor surgical outcomes grew longer; I do not miss adding additional names and images to this list. Those memories never disappeared or even diminished. Patient names and x-rays with good outcomes vanished from my memory bank without a trace, like names of distant cousins at a family reunion. But I could recite the names of patients whose cases did not have good outcomes.

I could draw up corpses from the memory graves of deformed limbs, of scary x-rays from gunshot wounds, of industrial accidents, and of motorcycle wrecks. I had hoped bad memories would someday decompose, but they haven't yet. Crushed left and right ankles of a drug-induced jump from a three-story building comes to mind, as well as the arm I had to amputate following a gunshot injury. I recall a sixteen-year-old who had waved his left arm out of a car window as an oncoming car sideswiped it and changed his life in an instant. I salvaged what I could. He is probably a grandparent by now.

After I'd been in practice for over a decade, I used to measure the quality of my life by questioning how satisfied I was at the end of the day compared to my early years in practice. Personal satisfaction and confidence had lurched along at times, but overall these traits increased as I moved through my career. I had grown more compassionate, had learned to be a better listener, and had raised the standard for my own satisfaction. But I always continued to understand orthopedics as what I did, not who I was.

The wealth of my life can be measured by the richness of my experiences. Throughout forty-three years of practice in orthopedic surgery, I tried not to give residents unsolicited advice, but I always managed to slip in, "If you can enjoy your career half as much as I have, you've got it made."

Although my license to practice did not change over the years, I continued to mature and learn. I appreciated Monaghan more and wished he were still around to provide advice and thought-provoking questions. My confidence improved as my opinions softened and relationships extended. What began as a job became a profession, and morphed into a calling.

~~~

I have lived through events both harrowing and splendid. Although my hair has turned gray with passing decades, the disappointing intensity of my last day of training in Kansas City has never diminished. I still recall my last afternoon with Monaghan with clarity and regret.

When I finished my last day of training in orthopedic surgery, my contract ended on a Friday but at no specified time. Mary and our two girls had moved two weeks earlier to Tulsa from Kansas City, and all my charts and paperwork had been completed for days. But at 3:30 p.m. on that last Friday, my VW still waited in the parking lot, packed and ready to go. And I was still with Monaghan.

"Let's have another cup of coffee for the road," said Monaghan. "I'll get it." Without saying so, my chief expected me to sit sipping cold coffee until five o'clock. He was aware my car was packed and sitting in the parking lot and that Mary was already waiting for me in Tulsa, but he never mentioned it.

That last cup of coffee was stout and one notch above room temperature.

As we sat in the lunchroom and I heard stories that contained no new information and little substance, I listened for a clue to be dismissed and get on the road—but there was none.

We sat in silence for several long minutes, Monaghan looking down at his coffee. He dragged his right index finger around the rim of his cup. "I'm going to miss you," he said in a low voice.

The statement startled me. I didn't know what to say, but I knew his words required a response. I said something like, "Yeah, me too."

As he retold more stories that I could have recited from memory, along with the pauses and exaggerations, I watched the wall clock's minute hand until it finally bumped to five o'clock over his left shoulder.

"My time is up," I tried to say in a casual manner as my feet shuffled me forward.

I stood first and initiated the handshake. He dragged his hand out of his pocket in slow motion and shook my hand. As I began walking to the hall door, I assumed he would walk the short distance with me, but I turned left down the empty hall by myself and passed two more rooms before I arrived at the main exit. I turned to look down that hall of memories toward the lunchroom. I didn't see him, but his shadow on the wall revealed he was still standing in the doorway to the hall.

The shadow moved, and he stepped into the hall where I could see him. With neither of us saying a word, he pulled his hand from his pocket, and keeping his hand at the same level, gave a weak wave of farewell—almost a slow flick of his wrist.

I wanted more.

I wanted more than a sip of cold coffee and a weak handshake on my last day of twelve years of grueling education. I wanted the last day in our orthopedic residents' program to represent not a single day, but a conclusion of over a decade of dedication: hundreds of books read, late night call-ins, relentless work shifts, endless lectures, and stress on family relationships. Instead, I shut my car door and drove away from my mentor and all those years of collected experience without one moment of intimacy shared between us.

~~~

Growing up in Muskogee, Oklahoma, the culture of the era had not included the intimacy of hugging. Men didn't hug other men—even male relatives—and I was lucky if I received a hug from a female relative. It just wasn't done in those days.

After I finished medical school, I was happy to see my mom hug my dad, but he didn't hug her back. I never saw him hug anyone. After my graduation ceremony, I hugged my father. He stood as straight as a soldier standing at attention. He didn't return the hug.

I wanted more.

Over the years I wondered at this lack of intimacy in the male culture, and at some stage in my maturation process, I took it upon myself to change it. I'd always hugged my children and Mary, but I began hugging extended family members, friends, and even patients when it was appropriate. During my medical training, no one had mentioned what was considered appropriate as far as hugging patients. Maybe it was an intuitive issue for other medical students, but it wasn't for me.

When I was young, tears filled my eyes when I heard "The Star-Spangled Banner" or experienced serious family events. But never, ever, would I have considered showing such emotion in a professional setting. And if I did begin to express genuine intimacy, where did it stop? Do I hug only the patient, if so, will the spouse feel left out? How do I handle the family after hugging the patient? If I hug more than one in the room would I be devaluing the patient?

I remember treating an elderly gentleman for a total knee replacement after he was involved in a terrible motor vehicle accident. His treatment stretched over eighteen months that were difficult for him and included four surgeries and extensive physical therapy. He made a satisfactory recovery, but at times the journey was overwhelming for him. I cared for him during those many months as he struggled with anxiety and depression.

At his last office visit we viewed his final x-rays together. I told him how well he was doing. We sat in silence, he on the exam table and me on a rolling stool. It was as if we had survived a battle together and neither of us knew what to say.

When I stood and moved toward him, he stood too and opened his arms. We held each other for a moment before I stepped back. When I did, I saw tears in his eyes.

"I've been wondering if you'd do that for me," he said. I nodded and smiled as a tear trailed down my cheek.

My experience with him taught me to read the mood and initiate a hug when a patient needed it. As my comfort level increased and I began to experience the profound shared joy of compassion and intimacy, I wished I'd started hugging patients earlier.

For so many years in my adult life, I would reach to hug my father and his arms would stay at his side. But gradually over the years he began bending his elbows as I approached to hug him, and I'd walk into his modified embrace, which was still not a hug. In his last years he finally squeezed my shoulders when I hugged him, but he still didn't pull me into his sphere of intimacy. Maybe that's why Monaghan's farewell during the last day of my residency left such an influential impression. I wanted to step into that shared circle of intimacy, compassion, and understanding with my mentor—and with my dad.

~~~

Years after I graduated from the residency program that had hardened my heart, I admitted many of the words that came out of my mouth belonged to Dr. Monaghan. Teaching personable, motivated young adults while maintaining a professional distance demanded that I straddle a thin gray line. I sent Monaghan a two-page thank you letter. In conclusion, I wrote:

> *From my exposure to you and by standing on your shoulders, the responsibility rests on me to pass these values to the orthopedic residents in our program. Procedures and issues evolve, but ethics and values do not. Because of your impact on me, I have much to pass to residents. You were my teacher and mentor. I open my mouth and your words come forth. The hours at Romano's were well spent. I thank you with love and appreciation.*
>
> *Love, Harold.*

Over the years of teaching, there was an issue I had determined from that disappointing ending with Monaghan. I would create a more expressive conclusion for each resident under my tutelage on his last day than my mentor had created for me. I vowed their last day would be meaningful, and I wished the idea had come to me earlier, but I was pleased with myself.

The first year I initiated my idea, I arranged for both graduating residents to be on my service their last day, but at different hours. When the first resident was leaving, I walked with him to his car and handed him a wrapped gift. He looked at me quizzically.

"What's this?"

"I guess you'll have to open it to find out," I said, shrugging my shoulders.

When he opened the box, he found twenty blank thank-you notes and twenty stamps.

"Who am I supposed to send these to?"

"You'll know when the time comes."

And then I delivered the kind of farewell I had always wanted to receive from my mentor and tutor, Dr. Monaghan—a goodbye hug of appreciation.

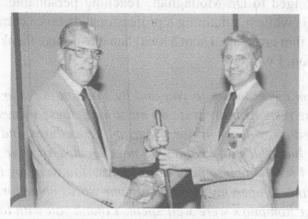

Dr. Monaghan   Dr. Battenfield

Acknowledgments

The following people have changed the trajectory of my life; my wife, Mary Battenfield; my orthopedic trainer, Dr. Monaghan; the forty-three orthopedic residents who graduated from our training program; trusting patients, caring friends, writing coaches and my editors – especially Stephanie Colburn, Sarah Stecher, Lauren King, and Grant King. To all I am grateful.

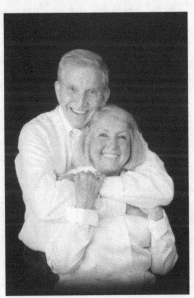

Harold and Mary

After Dr. Harold Battenfield retired from his career as an orthopedic surgeon in 2010, he returned to college and studied the art of writing—forty-three college hours—to better share his stories. In 2015 he published his first book, ***Braiding Generations: A Grandfather Breaks the***

Code. About those stories he wrote, "I choose to record mine in print to offer up what has been meaningful to me in life, so my children and grandkids can know their family history, become witnesses to who I am, and better understand what I think and feel. This is my story about what it means to be human."

And now in 2018 he offers us *Human Side of a Surgeon*, a book detailing his light and dark experiences as a medical student, his forty-one years of orthopedic practice, and his developing abilities as a teacher of those choosing careers in the profession he loved. These roles and events braided together and formed his character.

Forty-three orthopedic surgeons completed their training under the program he developed and nurtured. He also holds four medical patents.

Harold lives with his wife, Mary, in Tulsa, Oklahoma.

CPSIA information can be obtained
at www.ICGtesting.com
Printed in the USA
LVHW042142251019
635403LV00002B/36/P